Ernst Schering Foundation Symposium
Proceedings 2006-4
Immunotherapy in 2020

Ernst Schering Foundation Symposium
Proceedings 2006-4

Immunotherapy in 2020

Visions and Trends
for Targeting Inflammatory Disease

A. Radbruch, H.-D. Volk, K. Asadullah, W.-D. Doecke
Editors

With 10 Figures

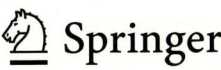 Springer

Series Editors: G. Stock and M. Lessl

Library of Congress Control Number: 2007928116

ISSN 0947-6075

ISBN 978-3-540-70850-6 Springer Berlin Heidelberg New York

Springer is a part of Springer Science+Business Media
springer.com

Editor: Dr. Ute Heilmann, Heidelberg
Desk Editor: Wilma McHugh, Heidelberg
Production Editor: Martin Weißgerber, Leipzig
Cover design: design & production, Heidelberg
Typesetting and production: LE-TEX Jelonek, Schmidt & Vöckler GbR, Leipzig
21/3180/YL – 5 4 3 2 1 0   Printed on acid-free paper

Preface

From 22 to 24 October 2006, internationally renowned scientists from the European Union and the United States met in Potsdam near Berlin, Germany, to discuss the future of chronic inflammatory disease treatment. The title of the symposium, organized by the Ernst Schering Foundation, was "Immunotherapy in 2020—Visions and Trends for Targeting Inflammatory Diseases".

The presentations covered the main mechanisms of immunoregulation such as peripheral and central tolerance, epigenetic programming, immunologic memory, and regulatory networks in inflammation as well as novel experimental and clinical approaches for targeting inflammation in autoimmunity and transplantation. Group discussions focused on the question of how recent findings in immunological research can lead to improved diagnostics, new drugs, and better therapies. In this regard, beside novel approaches, the individualization of immunomodulatory therapies and the establishment of reliable biomarkers for assessing the specific immune situation along with patient response to therapies were discussed.

In this volume, the symposium speakers give their view on current topics of immunopathophysiology and immunotherapy.

The chapter by Prof. Rikard Holmdahl (Section for Inflammation Research, Lund University, Sweden) deals with the genetic basis of inflammatory diseases by means of gene polymorphisms and its implications for the finding of new therapies. He describes how, based on the proven genetic component of rheumatoid arthritis demonstrated by clinical studies, a search for susceptibility genes in mice models was performed, which led to the definition of novel pathways involved in the immunopathology of arthritis. Concluding from this, novel therapeutic approaches are proposed which are experimentally proven yet.

The posttranscriptional networks in inflammation are the focus of the contribution from Dr. Dimitris Kontoyiannis and colleagues (Biomedical Sciences Research Center, Athens, Greece). The biosynthesis of inflammatory mediators relies on the biogenesis as well as the utilization of their corresponding mRNAs. These latter "utilization steps" encompass posttranscriptional mechanisms that impose a series of flexible rate-limiting controls to modify the abundance of a mRNA as well as its rate of translation to proteins. The chapter deals with RNA-binding proteins that, for example, by binding to the AU-rich family of elements, stringently control the maturation, localization, turnover, and translation of mRNAs from inflammatory genes.

Prof. Andreas Radbruch and colleagues (German Rheumatism Research Center, Berlin, Germany) give an up-to-date overview on immunological memory, its role in chronic inflammation, and its dramatic impact on the limitations of current immunotherapies. Concerning the latter, the humoral memory—which is provided by long-living plasma cells—is discussed in particular. The immunologic memory is not sufficiently targeted by current immunotherapies that suppress ongoing immune activation. This is probably one of the main reasons frustrating the cure of diseases by therapies, except bone marrow transplantation. Therefore, targeting of the immunologic memory, which provides a consistent trigger of relapse, might be a major challenge for future immunotherapies.

Adoptive T cell therapies are used to substitute the non-sufficient immune response of the recipient, e.g., to virus infection or malignancy. The use of unselective allogeneic T cell therapies (e.g., donor lymphocyte infusion), however, is limited by major clinical complications such as graft-versus-host disease. Dr. Stephen Gottschalk and colleagues (Center for Cell and Gene Therapy, Baylor College of Medicine, Houston, Texas, USA) deal with the development of autologous antigen-specific T cell therapies for the treatment of different Epstein-Barr virus-associated malignancies. If effective, these strategies might have broad implications also for other indications, e.g., human tumors with defined antigens.

Interesting novel perspectives of a rather old approach, polyclonal antibody therapy, are given in the contribution by Drs. Roland Buelow and Wim van Schooten (Therapeutic Human Polyclonals Inc., Mountain View, California, USA). Despite their strong development in the last few years (e.g., humanization, novel antibody derivatives, and conjugates), monoclonal antibody therapies have principal limitations. Hence, their effectiveness especially in devastating diseases such as cancer and infections is often limited by the capacity of single monoclonal antibodies to trigger immune effector functions as well as by the adaptivity of the affected cells and the pathogens (e.g., mutation or loss of antigen expression). These limitations of mono-specific antibodies might be overcome by therapeutic oligoclonal (mixtures of monoclonals) and polyclonal antibody preparations. A major step forward for the latter is the generation of human polyclonal antisera in transgenic animals.

The chapter by Prof. Hans-Dieter Volk and colleagues (Institute of Medical Immunology, Charité Hospital, Berlin, Germany) deals with a major challenge for all immunomodulatory interventions, the individualization of immunotherapy. By means of immunosuppressive and anti-infective therapy in transplant patients and patients with autoimmune disease, the authors describe how the patients can be selected for special adjuvant therapies, how the most suitable immunosuppression is selected for the single patient, and how the effect of a specific immunomodulatory therapy can be monitored to allow its timely adjustment to be sufficient while minimizing the side effects.

All in all, the meeting was characterized by very intensive and fruitful discussions involving the concepts and thinking of researchers from academia, pharmaceutical industry and clinics. There was agreement that only through the close cooperation of everyone involved in this research field a better understanding and finally a better immunotherapy for autoimmune diseases and allotransplantation can be achieved.

We would like to thank the Ernst Schering Foundation for sponsoring this meeting as well as all speakers and participants for their valuable input.

Andreas Radbruch
Hans-Dieter Volk
Khusru Asadullah
Wolf-Dietrich Doecke

Contents

List of Editors and Contributors

Editors

Radbruch, A.
Deutsches Rheuma-Forschungszentrum Berlin,
Schumanstr. 21/22, 10127 Berlin, Germany
(e-mail: radbruch@drfz.de)

Volk, H.-D.
Institute of Medical Immunology, Charité Campus Mitte,
Schumannstr. 20/21, 10117 Berlin, Germany
(e-mail: hans-dieter.volk@charite)

Asadullah, K.
Schering AG, Müllerstr. 178, 13342 Berlin, Germany
(e-mail: Khusru.Asadullah@bayerhealthcare.de)

Doecke, W.-D.
Schering AG, Müllerstr. 178, 13342 Berlin, Germany
(e-mail: Wolf-Dietrich.Doecke@bayerhealthcare.de)

Contributors

Albrecht, I.
Deutsches Rheuma-Forschungszentrum Berlin, Charitéplatz 1,
10117 Berlin, Germany
(e-mail: albrecht@drfz.de)

Bollard, C.M.
Center for Gene and Cell Therapy, Baylor College of Medicine,
6621 Fannin Street MC 3-3320, Houston, TX 77030, USA

Brenner, M.K.
Center for Gene and Cell Therapy, Baylor College of Medicine,
6621 Fannin Street MC 3-3320, Houston, TX 77030, USA

Buelow, R.
Therapeutic Human Polyclonals Inc, 2105 Landings Drive,
Mountain View, CA 94043, USA
(e-mail: roland@polyclonals.com)

Dimitriou, M.
BSRC "Alexander Fleming", Institute of Immunology, 34 A.
Fleming Str., Vari 16672, Greece

Dotti, G.
Center for Gene and Cell Therapy, Baylor College of Medicine,
6621 Fannin Street MC 3-3320, Houston, TX 77030, USA

Gottschalk, S.
Center for Gene and Cell Therapy, Baylor College of Medicine,
6621 Fannin Street MC 3-3320, Houston, TX 77030, USA
(e-mail: smg@bcm.edu)

Heslop, H.E.
Center for Gene and Cell Therapy, Baylor College of Medicine,
6621 Fannin Street MC 3-3320, Houston, TX 77030, USA

Holmdahl, R.
Medical Inflammation Research, Lund University, BMC I11,
221 84 Lund, Sweden
(e-mail: rikard.holmdahl@med.lu.se)

Katsanou, V.
BSRC "Alexander Fleming", Institute of Immunology, 34 A.
Fleming Str., Vari 16672, Greece

Kontoyiannis, D.L.
BSRC "Alexander Fleming", Institute of Immunology, 34 A.
Fleming Str., Vari 16672, Greece
(e-mail: d.kontoyiannis@fleming.gr)

Niesner, U.
Deutsches Rheuma-Forschungszentrum Berlin, Charitéplatz 1,
10117 Berlin, Germany
(e-mail: niesner@drfz.de)

Rooney, C.M.
Center for Gene and Cell Therapy, Baylor College of Medicine,
6621 Fannin Street MC 3-3320, Houston, TX 77030, USA

Savoldo, B.
Center for Gene and Cell Therapy, Baylor College of Medicine,
6621 Fannin Street MC 3-3320, Houston, TX 77030, USA

Schootem, W. v.
Therapeutic Human Polyclonals Inc, 2105 Landings Drive,
Mountain View, CA 94043, USA

Straathof, K.C.
Center for Gene and Cell Therapy, Baylor College of Medicine,
6621 Fannin Street MC 3-3320, Houston, TX 77030, USA

Ernst Schering Foundation Symposium Proceedings, Vol. 4, pp. 1–15
DOI 10.1007/2789_2007_036
© Springer-Verlag Berlin Heidelberg
Published Online: 15 June 2007

Nature's Choice of Genes Controlling Chronic Inflammation

R. Holmdahl(✉)

Medical Inflammation Research, I11 BMC, Lund University, 22184 Lund, Sweden
email: *rikard.holmdahl@med.lu.se*

Abstract. Inflammation is a physiological response that may go uncontrolled and thereby develop in a chronic way. This seems to happen in many common diseases of autoimmune, degenerative, or allergic character. Rheumatoid arthritis (RA) is by definition a chronic disease with an autoimmune inflammatory attack on diarthrodial cartilaginous joints. The development of new treatment neutralizing cytokines involved in the inflammatory attack has given relief and gives the promise of more effective treatment of already established disease. It is now time to set our eyes on a new vision to develop preventive and curative treatment based on knowledge of the unique and causative pathogenic mechanisms. To do this we believe it is important to identify the natural-selected polymorphisms that are associated with disease. These have proven to be extremely difficult to identify in complex diseases such as RA, but using animal models, this work is closer to reality. Animal models have recently been developed mimicking various aspects of the human disease. We will present an example in which a genetic polymorphism associated with the development of arthritis has been identified. On the basis of this finding, a new pathway involving control of immune tolerance by reactive oxidative species has been identified and a new class of antiinflammatory agents activating the induced oxidative burst protein complex is suggested.

1   Chronic Versus Acute Inflammation as Disease Mechanisms

There is a growing insight that inflammatory mechanisms are crucial in the molecular pathogenesis of many common diseases (Fig. 1). This is obvious in allergic diseases, which are caused by an exaggerated and disproportionate response to foreign antigens. These antigens are only partly known in conditions such as bronchial asthma. In another allergic disease, celiac disease, not only has the causative allergen been identified but also parts of the molecular pathways leading to disease (Sollid 2002). Clearly these diseases also involve autoimmune reactivities as a component of their pathology (Sollid and Jabri 2005). A second group of diseases comprises degenerative diseases, in which aberrant molecular structures or precipitates accumulate in tissue creating an inflammatory response. Some examples are atherosclerosis (Hansson and Libby 2006), adult onset macula degeneration (Nozaki et al. 2006), and Alzheimer disease (Wyss-Coray 2006). A third group is autoimmune diseases, in which autoimmune reactivates are believed to be the driving forces in the pathogenesis. Some examples are rheumatoid arthritis (RA), multiple sclerosis (MS), and type I diabetes. In all these diseases the inflammatory response needs to progress in a chronic and uncontrolled way to be regarded as pathogenic.

2   Rheumatoid Arthritis

RA is classified using a set of seven different criteria and it is essential that the disease manifest for at least 6 weeks (Fig. 2). In practice, patients have had clinical manifest disease for at least 1 year before they get the diagnosis, and they are still described as early RA. The classification criteria reflect the present knowledge and indicate the type of underlying inflammatory mechanisms (Fig. 2). Naturally the statistical

The pathogenic aberration in inflammatory diseases is chronic!

1) Autoimmune diseases; rheumatoid arthritis (RA), multiple sclerosis (MS), type I diabetes (T1D) etc
2) Degenerative diseases; spondyloarthropathies, atherosclerosis, Alzheimer, adult onset macula degeneration, osteoarthritis etc
3) Allergic diseases; Asthma bronchialis, chronic contact eczema, celiaki etc

But the inflammatory attack is iterative and acute!

Fig. 1. Grouping of inflammatory diseases

occurrence of RA is dependent on the diagnostic criteria used, but it is believed to be relatively common, affecting 0.5%–1% of the Caucasian population, and occurs worldwide (Symmons et al. 2002). Women are about three times more often affected by RA as compared to men. Genetically, both X and Y chromosomes could be of importance, but also autosomal chromosomes, as all genes interact with the context shaped by gender. One such context-shaping effect is mediated by sex steroids. However, it is a complex influence; the female sex steroids (estrogens) potently suppress T cell-dependent autoimmune diseases such as experimental arthritis, and it is likely that this is also the case in humans (Jansson and Holmdahl 1998). The clinical onset of RA seems to be very variable along the lifespan, but has a peak around 40–50 years of age, when estrogen levels drop. A typical example of development of RA would be a woman at the age of 50 that has had arthritis symptoms for a year before she is classified as having classical RA (Fig. 3). Her disease did not start, however, at the time of the onset of these symptoms; it most likely started years before. From analysis of historic blood samples, it is believed that formation of rheumatoid factors predicts the development of RA (Aho et al. 1985), and more recently it has been shown that this is also the case with antibodies to citrullinated proteins

(Rantapaa-Dahlqvist et al. 2003), which show high specificity for RA (Schellekens et al. 1998).

Monozygotic twin studies, with a concordance rate of approximately 15% and the heritability estimated to be 60% (MacGregor et al. 2000), indicate a significant but not prominent genetic component. It has however, been very difficult to identify the major genes in this complex disease. Hypothesis-free linkage analysis has not been able to significantly pinpoint any gene region apart from the major histocompatibility complex (MHC) region (John et al. 2006).

If genetic analysis is difficult, it is even more problematic to identify the environmental factors. An example of these difficulties arises in the many studies on the role of estrogen, which is consumed by a large part of the population (Bijlsma and van den Brink 1992). Some studies show a dramatic protective effect and some no effect at all. A proper metaanalysis showed no significant effect. It is likely that we will find some of the major genes before we find the major environmental factors.

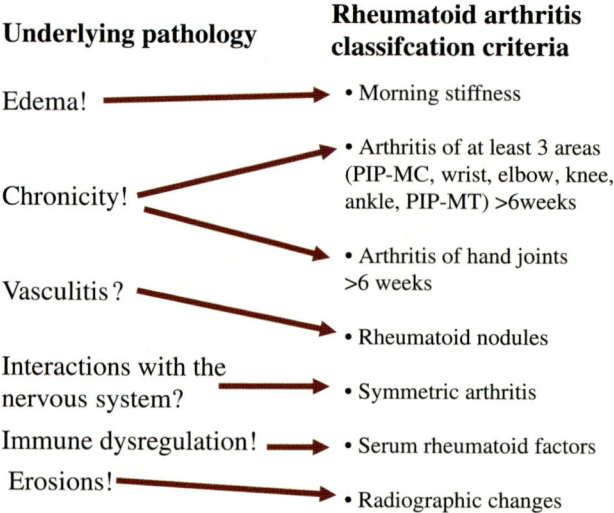

Fig. 2. The American Rheumatology Association classification criteria of RA and suggestions of the underlying pathology for each of the criteria

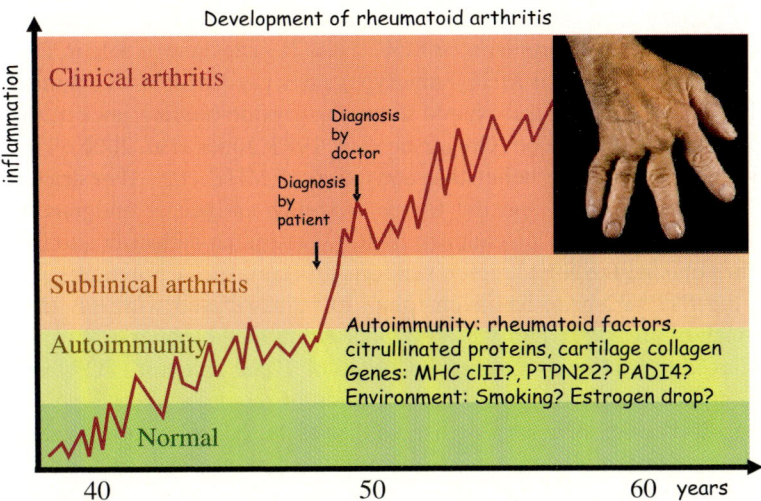

Fig. 3. A typical example of an untreated RA disease course. The disease activity is denoted "severity" on the y axis. Age is on the x axis. The curve represents an imaginary fluctuating disease activity of a woman developing RA. She is a smoker and carries an MHC haplotype expressing a shared epitope class II molecule. Maybe she has an RA-promoting PTPn22, PADI4, and other disease alleles. She develops rheumatoid factors and antibodies to citrullinated proteins starting even before symptoms of arthritis. When arthritis starts, it takes some time before she visits a rheumatologist and is given adequate treatment. The shown disease course is without effective treatment, as would have been the case some years ago, and she could expect a severe chronic relapsing disease and a premature death. Today she would have been given treatment, maybe with a combination of anti-TNFα and methotrexate, and the disease would have been less severe and less destructive

3   The MHC Region and Other RA Susceptibility Genes

An association between RA and the MHC region was observed a long time ago—before, in fact, the understanding of the fundamental function of MHC genes in the immune system (Stastny 1978). These data have subsequently been reproduced and refined in numerous studies in various populations. However, it has not yet been possible to identify the responsible gene, although circumstantial evidence strongly supports the idea that polymorphisms in MHC class II genes play a role in RA. It could be shown that MHC haplotypes associated with RA contained MHC class II genes that shared a similar peptide-binding pocket, the so-called shared epitope (Gregersen et al. 1987; Jones et al. 2006). This has given rise to the belief that activation of MHC class II restricted autoreactive T cells, specific for an unknown antigen or antigens, is a critical pathogenic mechanism in RA. Preliminary identification of genes outside the MHC region supports this concept. A polymorphism in the *PTPN22* gene has been found to be associated with RA (Begovich et al. 2004), and the functional effect of the polymorphism is believed to lead to a weaker association of T cell receptor (TCR) signaling and thereby less efficient activation of regulatory T cells (Vang et al. 2005). Another suggested candidate is the *PADI4* gene, encoding the enzyme peptidylarginine deiminase 4, which mediates the citrullination of proteins forming neoepitopes (Suzuki et al. 2003). However, we expect that these candidate genes only represent the tip of an iceberg containing hundreds of interacting genes. Higher statistical power and more controlled systems, such as animal models, are clearly necessary for more rapid progress on understanding the genetic control of RA.

4   Gene Searching Using Animal Models for RA

There has been an important development of new animal models for RA, and different models in the arsenal available today are likely to reflect several subtypes of RA. For studies of genetic control, the selected animal model not only needs to mimic RA as much as possible but also be highly reproducible and show different penetrance in different inbred strains. A useful model is pristane-induced arthritis (PIA) (Vingsbo et al. 1996). Pristane is an alkane with adjuvant properties that induces severe and chronic arthritis after injection of 150 µl in the back skin of DA (dark agouti) rats (Fig. 4). It fulfills the classification criteria for RA and is highly reproducible, reaching almost 100% incidence in DA, whereas some other strains such as E3 are completely resistant. Genetic mapping of genetically segregating cohorts at the second filial generation (F_2) levels has revealed about 20 quantitative trait loci

Pristane induced arthritis (PIA)

Induced with 150 µl pristane subcutaneously
2-4 weeks later: onset of severe polyarthritis

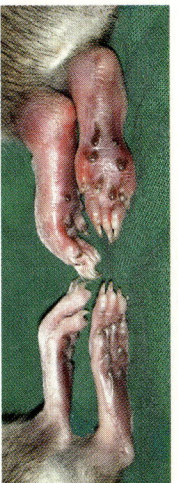

RA criteria	PIA
Morning stiffness	nd
Arthritis >3 areas, > 6 weeks	+
Arthritis hand, > 6 weeks	+
Symmetric arthritis	+
Rheumatoid noduli	nd
Serum rheumatoid factors	+
Joint erosions	+

CH₃
 |
CH- CH₂- CH₂- CH₂- CH- CH₂- CH₂- CH- CH₂- CH₂- CH₂- CH
 | | |
CH₃   CH₃   CH₃

Fig. 4. The pristane-induced arthritis (PIA) model is induced by a subcutaneous injection of 150 µl pristane (see indicated molecular structure). A chronic relapsing disease will develop fulfilling the criteria for classical RA

(QTLs) associated with the development of arthritis (Vingsbo-Lundberg et al. 1998). One QTLs determined in this way was the Pia4 locus on chromosome 12, which was associated with arthritis severity both during the acute and chronic relapsing periods.

5   Positional Cloning of Ncf1

The next step was to positionally clone the underlying genes responsible for this effect. This was done using the congenic approach (Olofsson et al. 2003). Thus the chromosomal fragment from the E3 strain containing the putative gene mediating protection against severe arthritis was moved into the DA background through ten repetitive backcrosses. Once the new congenic strain, DA.PIA4, had been established, it was tested and was found to develop only mild arthritis as compared with the DA littermates. The next step was to minimize the congenic fragment. To do this, we screened for new recombinants, and when we discovered them they were bred as new subcongenic strains and subsequently tested for arthritis susceptibility. At last a congenic strain—having only two genes in the E3-derived fragment—was found to protect against arthritis, and after sequencing and functional testing, it could be concluded that the responsible gene was *Ncf1*.

During this long-term project, this was in fact our last candidate gene, and the reason we excluded this gene from our list of possible candidates was that the allele that was associated with arthritis was also associated with lower oxidative burst, a phenomenon we, at that time, believed would promote inflammation and arthritis. However, we could at that point clearly show that an allele of *Ncf1*—coding for a protein (also named p47phox) with a structural polymorphism—was associated with a lower oxidative burst and also with more severe arthritis. To investigate a possible connection between these two phenomena, we needed another mutation in the *Ncf1* gene. In the rat it seemed that there was an extensive polymorphism of *Ncf1*, even in the wild population, but no other candidate mutation with the potential to show the same effect was discovered. We then searched in the mouse. In parallel genetic mapping studies in our laboratory, we had in fact isolated a locus around the *Ncf1* gene on chromosome 5 associated with experimental autoimmune encephalomyelitis (EAE) (Karlsson et al. 2003). However, after establishing the congenic strain we excluded *Ncf1* as a candidate, and we found the *Ncf1* gene is not as polymorphic in the mouse as it is in the rat. However, thanks to the work of Huang et al. (2000), we identified a B6 strain at the Jackson laboratories carrying a spontaneous *Ncf1* mutation. This mutation was backcrossed to the collagen-induced arthritis (CIA)-susceptible B10.Q strain, and we found that it dramatically reduced the capacity to make an oxidative burst. Testing this new strain with CIA clearly showed a similar phenotype as in the rat, and a severe chronic arthritis developed (Hultqvist et al. 2004). In fact, these mice could develop arthritis spontaneously during their postpartum period, a period known to be very sensitive to arthritis relapses due to the drop of estrogen (Mattsson et al. 1991). Interestingly, the autoantibody response to type II collagen (CII) was raised in the *Ncf1*-mutated mice. Thus we concluded that we had positionally cloned *Ncf1* as associated with arthritis severity, and that the genetically controlled pathway involved regulation of reactive oxidative species (ROS) production.

6   Functional Studies of Ncf1

NCF1 (alias p47phox) is a protein component of the nicotinamide adenine dinucleotide phosphate, reduced (NADPH) oxidase (NOX) complex, which is an inducer of oxidative burst into the extracellular compartment (Fig. 5). Using the established rat and mouse congenic strains, we had unique tools to investigate the role of this gene. First we could show that the disease associated with the *Ncf1* allele operated before or during T cell activation. This was done by transferring MHC class II-restricted CD4+ ab T cells between the DA and the DA.Pia4 rat (Olofsson et al. 2003). If the T cells originated from a DA.Pia4 donor, the protective E3 allele of *Ncf1* led to protection from arthritis in the recipient. Next we investigated whether the *Ncf1* gene was expressed in antigen-presenting cells or in the T cells. We found that several types of antigen-presenting cells, including macrophages and dendritic cells, expressed *Ncf1*, but not T cells. Thus, if T cell carries the information from the *Ncf1* gene, it needed to carry this information with a changed phenotype. To determine this phenotype we carefully investigated the

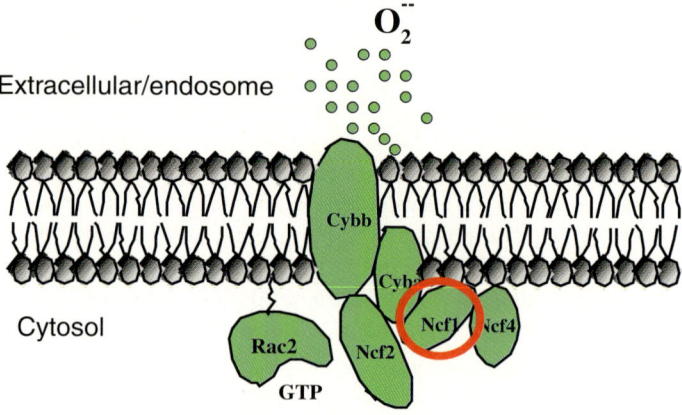

Fig. 5. The NADPH oxidase (NOX) complex showing the various subunits Ncf1 (p47phox), Ncf2 (p67phox), Ncf4 (40phox), Cybb (gp91), Cyba (gp20), and Rac2. When activated the complex releases oxygen radical anions to the outer space (extracellular or endosomal)

oxidative status of the T cells and found that T cells originating from DA rats had a lower number of thiol groups, i.e., free SH groups, on proteins in the cellular membrane as compared with T cells from DA.Pia4 rats (Gelderman et al. 2006). In contrast, no difference could be seen in the redox level of the cytosol. To determine whether the changed redox level in the cell membrane was responsible for the effect, we experimentally changed this by treating the cell in vitro with glutathione or with oxidized glutathione and then transferred them to nave recipients. The effect was clear: oxidation of the T cell membrane led to less arthritis and reduction of the T cell membrane to enhanced arthritis. Likewise, reduced T cells survived better in vivo and migrated to the to the joints. Thus we had identified at least one of the molecular pathways explaining the genetic effect. We suggest that T cells were educated, presumably by interacting with antigen-presenting cells, through exposure of ROS, leading to changed redox levels of their T cell membranes (Fig. 6). If correct, this finding will have implications not only for understanding arthritis, but also for T cell selection, tolerance, and immunity.

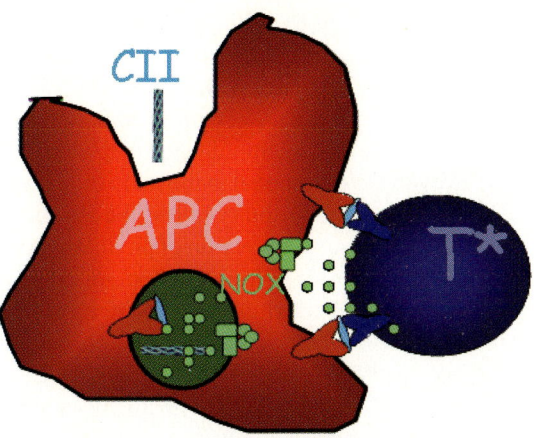

Fig. 6. A hypothetical model showing ROS as transmitters. An antigen-presenting cell (*APC*) could be a dendritic cell or a macrophage that express *NCF1* and have a functional NOX complex. The APC takes up type II collagen (*CII*) and processes it in the endosomes, and peptides are bound to the MHC class II molecules. Costimulatory agents will activate the NOX complex in the endosomal membrane and in the lipid rafts on the cell surface. They will oxidize the endosomal lumen as well as the synapse formed between the APC and the interacting antigen-specific T cell. Here the produced ROS will act as a transmitter produced by the APC and acting on the T cell surface

7   Ncf1 as a Pharmacologic Target

If activation of the *Ncf1*-containing NOX complex has such an important role in T cell autoimmunity and in regulating arthritis, it should serve as a possible target candidate for antiinflammatory treatment. Thus we developed a quite extensive program to identify substances that could activate the NOX complex and induce an enhanced oxidative burst capacity in vivo. As a prototype compound we selected synthetic phytol, a naturally occurring hydrocarbon (Hultqvist et al. 2006). Subcutaneous injection of phytol in DA rats led to a restoration of the low oxidative burst capacity within 24 h. One injection in fact gave a relatively long-lasting effect of 4–5 weeks. Importantly, treated rats developed an almost complete protection against arthritis.

To be of value for treating an already established chronic disease, the compound also needed to be tested in a relevant chronic phase of the disease. This is in fact seldom done, as there are few RA models with a chronic relapsing disease course. Normally, validation in the animal models is made only by preventing immune priming or possibly the onset of arthritis. However, the PIA model in the rat is truly chronic relapsing, which gave us a unique opportunity to test the chronic phase. The result was very promising: a single injection of phytol treatment stopped the progression of the disease for at least 4 weeks. Interestingly, phytol treatment of collagen-induced arthritis was also effective. In this model the autoimmune response could be evaluated, and phytol treatment led to a similar effect as a protective *Ncf1* allele; both the T cell-dependent autoantibody response to CII and delayed-type hypersensitive reactions were reduced, arguing that phytol affected the same T cell modulatory oxidative pathways as *Ncf1*.

8   Conclusion

Finding genes controlling complex diseases has not been an easy task, but the example of the positional cloning of *Ncf1* shows that it is possible. The *Ncf1* polymorphism is naturally selected and has profound effects on the control of both T cell autoimmunity and the development of chronic autoimmune inflammation as in arthritis. Isolation of the polymorphism in congenic strains also gives relevant in vivo tools to investigate the functional role of the gene in a complex contextual setting. We found that reactive oxidative species regulate T cell activation through oxidizing the thiol groups in the T cell membrane. We hypothesize that ROS are transmitters in the immunological synapse and regulate the activation threshold of T cell activation. The immune-activation outcome is thereby regulated by the involved antigen-presenting cell, and such a mechanism might be fundamental as an operative in all interactions between antigen-presenting cells and T cells.

Acknowledgements. I am grateful for support from several foundations that have made this work possible: the Anna Greta Crafoord, King Gustaf V:s 80-year, the Swedish Science Research Council, the Strategic Research Foundation, and the EU project NeuroproMiSe—LSHM-CT-2005-018637 and LSHM-CT-2005-005223 (Euraps).

References

Aho K, Palosuo T, Raunio V, Puska P, Aromaa A, Salonen JT (1985) When does rheumatoid disease start? Arthritis Rheum 28:485–489

Begovich AB, Carlton VE, Honigberg LA, Schrodi SJ, Chokkalingam AP, Alexander HC, Ardlie KG, Huang Q, Smith AM, Spoerke JM, Conn MT, Chang M, Chang SY, Saiki RK, Catanese JJ, Leong DU, Garcia VE, McAllister LB, Jeffery DA, Lee AT, Batliwalla F, Remmers E, Criswell LA, Seldin MF, Kastner DL, Amos CI, Sninsky JJ, Gregersen PK (2004) A missense single-nucleotide polymorphism in a gene encoding a protein tyrosine phosphatase (PTPN22) is associated with rheumatoid arthritis. Am J Hum Genet 75:330–337

Bijlsma JW, van den Brink HR (1992) Estrogens and rheumatoid arthritis. Am J Reprod Immunol 28:231–234

Gelderman KA, Hultqvist M, Holmberg J, Olofsson P, Holmdahl R (2006) T-cell surface redox levels determine T-cell reactivity and arthritis susceptibility. Proc Natl Acad Sci USA 103:12831–12836

Gregersen PK, Silver J, Winchester RJ (1987) The shared epitope hypothesis. An approach to understanding the molecular genetics of susceptibility to rheumatoid arthritis. Arthritis Rheum 30:1205–1213

Hansson GK, Libby P (2006) The immune response in atherosclerosis: a double-edged sword. Nat Rev Immunol 6:508–519

Huang CK, Zhan L, Hannigan MO, Ai Y, Leto TL (2000) P47(phox)-deficient NADPH oxidase defect in neutrophils of diabetic mouse strains, C57BL/6J-m db/db and db/+. J Leukoc Biol 67:210–215

Hultqvist M, Olofsson P, Holmberg J, Backstrom BT, Tordsson J, Holmdahl R (2004) Enhanced autoimmunity, arthritis, and encephalomyelitis in mice with a reduced oxidative burst due to a mutation in the Ncf1 gene. Proc Natl Acad Sci USA 101:12646–12651

Hultqvist M, Olofsson P, Gelderman KA, Holmberg J, Holmdahl R (2006) A new arthritis therapy with oxidative burst inducers. PLoS Med 3:e348

Jansson L, Holmdahl R (1998) Estrogen-mediated immunosuppression in autoimmune diseases. Inflamm Res 47:290–301

John S, Amos C, Shephard N, Chen W, Butterworth A, Etzel C, Jawaheer D, Seldin M, Silman A, Gregersen P, Worthington J (2006) Linkage analysis of rheumatoid arthritis in US and UK families reveals interactions between HLA-DRB1 and loci on chromosomes 6q and 16p. Arthritis Rheum 54:1482–1490

Jones EY, Fugger L, Strominger JL, Siebold C (2006) MHC class II proteins and disease: a structural perspective. Nat Rev Immunol 6:271–282

Karlsson J, Zhao X, Lonskaya I, Neptin M, Holmdahl R, Andersson A (2003) Novel quantitative trait loci controlling development of experimental autoimmune encephalomyelitis and proportion of lymphocyte subpopulations. J Immunol 170:1019–1026

MacGregor AJ, Snieder H, Rigby AS, Koskenvuo M, Kaprio J, Aho K, Silman AJ (2000) Characterizing the quantitative genetic contribution to rheumatoid arthritis using data from twins. Arthritis Rheum 43:30–37

Mattsson R, Mattsson A, Holmdahl R, Whyte A, Rook GA (1991) Maintained pregnancy levels of oestrogen afford complete protection from post-partum exacerbation of collagen-induced arthritis. Clin Exp Immunol 85:41–47

Nozaki M, Raisler BJ, Sakurai E, Sarma JV, Barnum SR, Lambris JD, Chen Y, Zhang K, Ambati BK, Baffi JZ, Ambati J (2006) Drusen complement components C3a and C5a promote choroidal neovascularization. Proc Natl Acad Sci USA 103:2328–2333

Olofsson P, Holmberg J, Tordsson J, Lu S, Akerstrom B, Holmdahl R (2003) Positional identification of Ncf1 as a gene that regulates arthritis severity in rats. Nat Genet 33:25–32

Rantapaa-Dahlqvist S, de Jong BA, Berglin E, Hallmans G, Wadell G, Stenlund H, Sundin U, van Venrooij WJ (2003) Antibodies against cyclic citrullinated peptide and IgA rheumatoid factor predict the development of rheumatoid arthritis. Arthritis Rheum 48:2741–2749

Schellekens GA, de Jong BA, van den Hoogen FH, van de Putte LB, van Venrooij WJ (1998) Citrulline is an essential constituent of antigenic determinants recognized by rheumatoid arthritis-specific autoantibodies. J Clin Invest 101:273–281

Sollid LM (2002) Coeliac disease: dissecting a complex inflammatory disorder. Nat Rev Immunol 2:647–655

Sollid LM, Jabri B (2005) Is celiac disease an autoimmune disorder? Curr Opin Immunol 17:595–600

Stastny P (1978) Association of the B-cell alloantigen DRw4 with rheumatoid arthritis. N Engl J Med 298:869–871

Suzuki A, Yamada R, Chang X, Tokuhiro S, Sawada T, Suzuki M, Nagasaki M, Nakayama-Hamada M, Kawaida R, Ono M, Ohtsuki M, Furukawa H, Yoshino S, Yukioka M, Tohma S, Matsubara T, Wakitani S, Teshima R, Nishioka Y, Sekine A, Iida A, Takahashi A, Tsunoda T, Nakamura Y, Yamamoto K (2003) Functional haplotypes of PADI4, encoding citrullinating enzyme peptidylarginine deiminase 4, are associated with rheumatoid arthritis. Nat Genet 34:395–402

Symmons D, Turner G, Webb R, Asten P, Barrett E, Lunt M, Scott D, Silman A (2002) The prevalence of rheumatoid arthritis in the United Kingdom: new estimates for a new century. Rheumatology (Oxford) 41:793–800

Vang T, Congia M, Macis MD, Musumeci L, Orru V, Zavattari P, Nika K, Tautz L, Tasken K, Cucca F, Mustelin T, Bottini N (2005) Autoimmune-associated lymphoid tyrosine phosphatase is a gain-of-function variant. Nat Genet 37:1317–1319

Vingsbo C, Sahlstrand P, Brun JG, Jonsson R, Saxne T, Holmdahl R (1996) Pristane-induced arthritis in rats: a new model for rheumatoid arthritis with a chronic disease course influenced by both major histocompatibility complex and non-major histocompatibility complex genes. Am J Pathol 149:1675–1683

Vingsbo-Lundberg C, Nordquist N, Olofsson P, Sundvall M, Saxne T, Pettersson U, Holmdahl R (1998) Genetic control of arthritis onset, severity and chronicity in a model for rheumatoid arthritis in rats. Nat Genet 20:401–404

Wyss-Coray T (2006) Inflammation in Alzheimer disease: driving force, bystander or beneficial response? Nat Med 12:1005–1015

Ernst Schering Foundation Symposium Proceedings, Vol. 4, pp. 17–35
DOI 10.1007/2789_2007_037
© Springer-Verlag Berlin Heidelberg
Published Online: 15 June 2007

Targeting of Memory

U. Niesner, I. Albrecht, A. Radbruch(✉)

Deutsches Rheuma-Forschungszentrum Berlin, Schumannstr. 21/22,
10117 Berlin, Germany
email: *radbruch@drfz.de*

Abstract. Current therapeutic options that are based on immunosuppression do not provide a cure for the treatment of chronic inflammation. Though more efficient immunosuppression and the introduction of biologicals such as antibodies targeting cytokines have improved clinical outcomes, immunosuppressive therapy has to be continued to be efficient, thus enhancing the risk of adverse events and undesired side effects. Why can immunosuppression ameliorate, even stop, but not cure chronic inflammation? Is chronic inflammation perpetuated beyond suppression by mechanisms independent of the immune system, or is it perpetuated by components of the immune system which are resistant to a block of ongoing immune reactions? One such component of the immune system is immunological memory. This article will review the role of immunological memory in chronic inflammation, as far as we understand it today, and discuss implications for the development of novel therapeutic strategies aiming at a cure for diseases involving chronic inflammation.

1 Immunological Memory and Chronic Inflammation

Immunological memory is a hallmark of the adaptive immune response. It is dependent on a dialog between T and B lymphocytes recognizing the antigens. T helper (Th) lymphocytes provide the critical signals for the generation of memory B and T lymphocytes. The heterogeneity of memory lymphocytes resembles the functional diversity of lymphocytes in general, with regulatory, helper, and effector T lymphocytes; B lymphocytes expressing antigen-receptors, which are affinity-matured and class switched; and plasma cells, which secrete such antibodies (Lanzavecchia and Sallusto 2005; Kalia et al. 2006; Radbruch et al. 2006). Upon rechallenge with the antigen, memory B and T lymphocytes will react faster and their reaction will be functionally imprinted, i.e., independent of the physiological (and therapeutic influenceable) regulation of primary immune responses (Lohning et al. 2002). Apart from this reactive immunological memory, long-lived plasma cells, and probably also effector memory T cells, can secrete antibodies and cytokines, respectively, without proliferation, and thus are resistant to all therapies targeting proliferating cells, e.g., corticosteroids (Miller 1964; Brinkmann and Kristofic 1995), γ-irradiation (Slifka 1998; Grayson et al. 2002), and cyclophosphamide (Orme 1988; Hoyer et al. 2004).

Chronic inflammation is an essential pathogenetic element of many diseases such as rheumatoid arthritis (RA), type 1 diabetes, multiple sclerosis, systemic lupus erythematosus (SLE), spondyloarthropathies, asthma, psoriasis, and inflammatory bowel disease. Although variable, the genetic component of such diseases has been estimated to be not more than 30%, with, for instance, more than 30 different genes possibly being involved in RA. This genetic heterogeneity is reflected by the diversity of clinical progress and responsiveness to treatment.

Inflammatory diseases commonly progress through distinct phases, with long periods of subclinical disease progression into a relapse/remitting or chronic-progressive inflammatory, clinically apparent phenotype. In general, at diagnosis the disease has already progressed to the chronic phase. Retrospective analyses of patients with RA have shown a break of tolerance to self and the development of a humoral memory of secreted antibodies to self (rheumatoid factor) or modified self (citrullinated peptides) preceding treatment by up to 10 years. In combination with genetic predisposition, e.g., the human leukocyte antigen (HLA)-DR4 "shared epitope," and environmental factors, e.g., tobacco smoking, the presence of such autoantibodies is a strong predictor of disease (Rantapaa-Dahlqvist et al. 2003; Klareskog et al. 2004). Currently, it can only be speculated that excessive immune reactions to pathogens might result in a break of tolerance and the generation of an immunological memory response to self in humans. Likewise, we have no information to date on how an acute, pathogen-driven inflammation is converted into a chronic inflammation which presumably is driven by self antigens. Current concepts are derived from animal models, demonstrating that such mechanisms could operate in principle. In particular, studies on the pathogenesis of the lupus-like disease in NZB/W mice have shown that an immunological memory of secreted antibodies specific for self antigens, e.g., DNA, is generated very early in ontogeny. Later in disease development, chronic immune reactions dominate, while the humoral memory for self persists. Moreover, it could be shown that this humoral memory is resistant to strong immunosuppression by cyclophosphamide, while the chronic immune reaction is completely abolished by this treatment (Hoyer et al. 2004).

A key question for assessing the role of immunological memory in the chronic phase of inflammation is whether or not (auto)immunity in the chronic phase is driven by (auto)antigen. The (auto)antigen-dependent case would be indicated by the reactivation of memory B and T cells, and their differentiation into effector cells, which in turn could be either short-lived or long-lived. The antigen-independent case would be indicated by the reactivation of memory B and T cells by pathogen-associated molecular patterns (PAMP) and/or cytokines. It has been elegantly demonstrated that memory B lymphocytes are readily activated into antibody-secreting cells by PAMP such as CpG-containing DNA and cytokines (Bernasconi et al. 2002). Whether or not these antibody-secreting cells have the potential to become long-lived remains to be shown. The antigen-independent case would also be indicated by the secretion of (auto)antibodies by long-lived plasma cells, i.e., the humoral memory. And for murine T memory cells, antigen-independent secretion of the cytokine interferon(IFN)-γ, a cytokine of key relevance for the regulation of inflammation, has been described (Yang et al. 2001).

Today we do not yet have clear proof that immunological memory is the missing target in our quest for a cure of chronic inflammation. Chronic inflammation persists through immunosuppression and provides secreted autoantibodies in the absence of the original antigenic trigger. It remains to be shown whether or not these autoantibodies suffice to perpetuate inflammation beyond immunosuppression. At present, the best evidence is provided by the experimental therapy of complete immunoablation in patients with autoimmune diseases such as SLE, juvenile idiopathic arthritis, or multiple sclerosis (Rosen et al. 2000; De Kleer et al. 2004; Jayne et al. 2004; Muraro et al. 2005; Tyndall and Saccardi 2005). Ablative protocols depleting memory, in particular long-lived, autoantibody-secreting plasma cells, have been curative in patients who had not responded to efficient immunosuppression. Their new immune system, generated from stem cells, was tolerant against those antigens to which they had reacted before.

2 Reactive Memory

2.1 T Cell Memory

Th cells, in particular T helper type 1 (Th1) and Th17 cells, are potent inducers of inflammation. This has been demonstrated in murine models of multiple sclerosis (Lafaille et al. 1997; Langrish et al. 2005), RA (Murphy et al. 2003; Maffia et al. 2004), and inflammatory bowel disease (Iqbal et al. 2002; Yen et al. 2006). Th1 cells, defined by the expression of IFN-γ, promote activation and recruitment of phagocytic cells and the B cell switch to complement-fixing IgG antibodies, such as IgG1 in humans. IFN-γ facilitates the homing of Th1 cells and B cells into inflamed tissues by inducing expression of the C-X-C motif chemokine receptor 3 (CXCR3) and its ligands CXCL-9, CXCL-10, and CXCL-11 (Nakajima et al. 2002; Rotondi et al. 2003; Muehlinghaus et al. 2005). Th17 cells secreting interleukin (IL)-17 activate fibroblasts, neutrophils, and epithelial cells to express a wide range of inflammatory mediators such as matrix metalloproteinases, CXCL-1, CXCL-8, IL-6, TNF-α, and IL-1β (Kolls and Linden 2004).

It has been amply demonstrated that Th1 and Th17 cells can induce inflammation in rodent models of inflammation. It is less clear, however, whether they also drive inflammation in the chronic phase of inflammation. Memory Th cells constitute a significant proportion of the cellular infiltrate present in chronically inflamed tissue, such as the synovium of inflamed joints in RA (Thomas et al. 1992). In particular, terminally differentiated memory cells, i.e., CD45RA–/CD27– Th cells (Kohem et al. 1996), which probably had been repeatedly stimulated, are frequent in inflamed synovia. Functionally, many of these cells are imprinted to re-express IL-17 or IFN-γ. The levels of IL-17 and IFN-γ are enhanced in the inflamed joints (Ziolkowska et al. 2000), and many T cell clones derived from inflamed tissue of RA patients have a memory for the expression of IL-17 and IFN-γ (Morita et al. 1998; Aarvak et al. 1999).

As part of the reactive memory, Th memory cells could fuel a chronic inflammation, either upon reactivation by (auto)antigen, or independent of T cell receptor stimulation, by cytokines and ligands of pattern-recognition receptors, both provided by the micro environment in the lesion (Cope 2002; Brennan et al. 2006). The latter, antigen-independent activation of Th1 memory cells has been shown to induce them to secrete IFN-γ, even over extended periods of time (Yang et al. 2001). It is less clear if other cytokines can be expressed by Th memory cells activated independent of their antigen. Although in RA particular HLA class II alleles are associated with poor prognosis, i.e., a more progressive joint destruction (Calin et al. 1989), the contribution of antigen-dependent activation of memory Th cells to the perpetuation of inflammation remains unclear so far.

Another critical role for reactive memory Th cells in the pathogenesis of inflammation and its perpetuation is their essential help for the differentiation of B cells into long-lived plasma cells, secreting (auto)antibodies of enhanced affinity and switched isotype, at least in diseases with (auto)antibody-driven pathogenesis of chronic inflammation such as SLE. In the K/BxN murine model of RA, Th cells, despite their instrumental role in initiation of disease, are even dispensable later, in the chronic phase. In these mice, Th cells are required initially for the induction of autoreactive, presumably long-lived plasma cells that produce arthritogenic autoantibodies and drive the later stages of the disease, then are independent of further contributions of T cells (Korganow et al. 1999).

So far, therapeutic targeting of Th cells in the context of chronic inflammatory diseases has been rather discouraging. Systemic depletion of Th cells by antibodies directed against CD4 showed some initial clinical benefit (Horneff et al. 1991; Choy et al. 1996). However, the approach had to be abandoned due to the lack of efficacy, and concerns regarding the immunodeficiency induced. Immunomodulatory, nondepleting anti-CD3 and anti-CD4 antibodies aiming at the selective inhibition of pathogenic T cell responses and at the same time boosting the T cell-dependent regulatory mechanisms are under investigation (Nepom 2002; Panaccione et al. 2005). Future studies will reveal the potential of this approach, although expectations have been dampened by the lack of success using a superagonistic anti-CD28 antibody (Suntharalingam et al. 2006).

Apart from Th lymphocytes, the relevance of $CD8^+$ cytotoxic T cells for the initiation and, in particular, for the perpetuation of chronic inflammation remains elusive. The strong genetic predisposition of MHC class I antigen HLA-B27 for ankylosing spondylitis (Brewerton et al. 1973) points to an important role of the MHC class I-dependent $CD8^+$ cells in this disease. Murine models of chronic inflammatory diseases differ in their dependency on $CD8^+$ T cells. $CD8^+$ T cells mediate diabetes in the NOD mouse strain (DiLorenzo and Serreze 2005), while CD8 T cells are dispensable for the induction of collagen-induced arthritis, or are antiinflammatory (Ehinger et al. 2001; Taneja et al. 2002).

2.2   B Cell Memory

Memory B cells accumulate in inflamed tissue as a result of immigration and local expansion (Schroder et al. 1996). In the past few years, B cells have been receiving increasing attention as mediators and regulators of chronic inflammation. This interest has been essentially fuelled by the remarkable efficacy of B cell-depleting therapies in established RA and SLE. Rituximab, a chimerized monoclonal antibody recognizing CD20, a surface molecule that is expressed by various B cell subsets except plasma cells, has been successfully used in the treatment of SLE (Leandro et al. 2005; Smith et al. 2006) and RA (Cohen et al. 2006; Emery et al. 2006).

B cells can contribute to the development and perpetuation of chronic inflammation in multiple ways. Memory B cells are potent antigen-presenting cells of their cognate antigen, they secrete proinflammatory cytokines, and they can fuel immune responses with the aberrant production of pathogenic antibodies in particular autoantibodies upon differentiation into plasma cells. That several of those effects can play a role simultaneously in an inflammatory context has been demonstrated in lupus-prone MRL/*lpr* mice. In these mice, B cells contribute to the development of lethal immunopathology by the production of pathologic autoantibodies and by antibody-independent mechanisms. B cell-deficient mice (MRL-JHd) fail to develop autoimmune manifestations, e.g., vasculitis and nephritis (Chan et al. 1999), while mice in which the B cells are incapable of secreting antibodies (MRL/*lpr* mIgM) do develop lethal autoimmune manifestations even while mortality is reduced by 50% (Chan et al. 1999).

A possible explanation for the antibody-independent mechanisms of B cell action is their role as potent antigen-presenting cells. Memory B cells efficiently present antigen to Th cells in an inflammatory context via MHC class II, thereby activating Th cells to proliferate and release proinflammatory cytokines (Roosnek and Lanzavecchia 1991; Roth et al. 1996; Falcone et al. 1998). In particular they do express B7h, the ligand for inducible costimulator (ICOS), and thus can efficiently costimulate ICOS[+] Th cells, which have been shown to be essential for induction of chronic inflammation (Lohning et al. 2003).

However, just as memory T cells can be activated in an antigen-independent way, the same holds true for memory B cells. Human memory B cells express pattern-recognition receptors such as the Toll-like receptors 6 (TLR-6), -7, -9, and -10 that are absent or only weakly expressed by naïve B cells (Bernasconi et al. 2003). They display a lower threshold of activation compared to naïve B cells and do not require further T cell help for activation and differentiation into antibody-secreting cells. "Rheumatoid factors" are low-affinity autoreactive antibodies targeting autologous antibodies, and their presence indicates development of RA. Autoreactive B cells with the capability to produce such autoantibodies might be activated independent of T cell help by antibody–RNA or antibody–chromatin immune complexes crosslinking the antibody-specific B cell receptor and TLR-7, or TLR-9, respectively (Leadbetter et al. 2002; Lau et al. 2005). Furthermore, in combination with TLR ligand stimulation, cytokines might substitute for B cell receptor signaling, leading to a polyclonal activation of memory B cells and differentiation into antibody-secreting cells (Bernasconi et al. 2003).

3   Humoral Memory

Humoral immunity can be provided by long-lived antibody-secreting plasma cells that maintain protective antibody titers following termination of the immune reaction, or by short-lived antibody-secreting cells that are constantly generated in a chronic immune reaction (Radbruch et al. 2006). Antigen bound to secreted antibodies triggers a multitude of effector functions through the constant region of the antibody heavy chains. This can contribute essentially to immunopathology already in otherwise protective immune reactions, but even more so in autoreactive immune responses. Secreted autoreactive antibodies are one of the mechanisms with the potential to fuel chronicity of inflammation. Autoantibodies can block or stimulate signaling pathways upon binding and crosslinking of cell-surface receptors (Drachman 1994; Chistiakov 2003). Deposition of immune complexes, i.e., antibody-antigen complexes, and opsonization of cellular or extracellular matrix structures at the site of inflammation or initially unaffected tissue leads to activation of complement and Fc-receptor-bearing phagocytic cells. This results in the release of proinflammatory mediators and ultimately in destruction of the surrounding tissue and organ failure, e.g., kidney destruction in SLE. In addition, immune complexes represent a continuous source of antigen and costimulation for activation of more autoreactive B and T cells. Autoantibodies specific for particular autoantigens are a hallmark of many autoimmune diseases. Their specificities range from cellsurface molecules, e.g., antiacetylcholine receptor in myasthenia gravis (Drachman 1994) to intracellular and nuclear antigens, e.g., antinuclear antibodies in SLE, or low-affinity anti-IgG (rheumatoid factor) in RA. They also can be specific for products of inflammation such as citrullinated peptides. Specificity, affinity, isotype, and concentration of autoantibodies are valuable diagnostic tools with considerable prognostic value (Dorner and Hansen 2004). High titers of rheumatoid factor, and antibodies recognizing citrullinated peptides are predictive for a more aggressive erosive disease course in RA (Vencovsky et al. 2003; Dorner and Hansen 2004; Machold et al. 2006).

Antibodies are produced by plasmablasts and by plasma cells that differentiate from any type of B cell upon antigenic stimulation and appropriate costimulatory signals (Radbruch et al. 2006). This differentiation step is fundamental; it is controlled by a switch of transcriptional programs regulated by paired box protein 5 (Pax5) in B cells, versus B lymphocyte-induced maturation protein 1 (Blimp1) and X-box binding protein 1 (XBP1) in antibody-secreting cells. Plasma cells are nondividing, have lost surface expression of MHC class II and antibody, as well as CD20, i.e., they are resistant to CD20-directed therapy with rituximab. The lifetime of plasma cells depends on their environment. Survival niches for plasma cells are found in the bone marrow, but also in inflamed tissue. Accordingly, plasma cells are enriched in chronically inflamed tissue such as the inflamed synovium of RA patients (Tsubaki et al. 2005) and the inflamed lamina propria of patients suffering from inflammatory bowel disease (Keren et al. 1987). Proinflammatory mediators present at sites of inflammation, such as TNF-α, IL-6, CXCL-12, and ligands for CD44, have been shown *in vitro* to support survival of plasma cells (Minges Wols et al. 2002; Cassese et al. 2003). In lupus-prone NZB/W mice, plasma cells that are generated early in the disease, before 12 weeks of age, form a pool of long-lived plasma cells and are resistant to immunosuppression by cyclophosphamide. These cells reside in the bone marrow and also in the spleen. Interestingly, later in the course of disease, such long-lived plasma cells no longer develop. Instead, short-lived plasmablasts and plasma cells are generated by chronic activation of B cells, a process that can be stopped by cyclophosphamide (Hoyer et al. 2004).

The coexistence of short-lived and long-lived plasma cells secreting autoreactive antibodies could also explain the differential effect of anti-CD20 therapy (rituximab) on titers of autoantibodies versus protective antibodies in patients with rheumatic diseases. The depletion of peripheral B cells, i.e., plasma cell precursors, should affect mainly the generation of short-lived plasma cells, while long-lived plasma cells should be resistant to rituximab. In RA patients, the titers of protective, tetanus or diphtheria-specific antibodies remain constant upon rituximab treatment, while the titers of disease-related autoantibodies specific for cit-rullinated proteins and rheumatoid factor drop significantly to levels that might indicate the proportion of autoantibodies secreted by long-lived plasma cells (Cambridge et al. 2003; Edwards et al. 2004). It should be noted that long-lived plasma cells could also be indirectly targeted by rituximab, if their survival niches in inflamed tissue would be resolved by amelioration of inflammation. Only long-lived plasma cells of the bone marrow should be completely resistant to rituximab.

The exact role of autoantibodies provided by long-lived plasma cells in the pathogenesis of chronic inflammatory disorders remains to be elucidated, but the autoantibodies are an elegant explanation for the long periods of subclinical disease progression, refraction to immuno-suppression, relapse upon termination of immunosuppression, and pre-vention of cure by currently available therapeutic strategies. Long-lived plasma cells memorize autoreactivity in the face of immunosuppression.

4   Current Immunosuppressive Therapies Do Not Provide a Cure

Today, therapeutic management of chronic inflammation relies on long-term immunosuppression. With more tailored regimens and combina-tion therapies, patients suffering from chronic inflammatory disorders nowadays can expect clear-cut and long-lasting amelioration of disease symptoms, reduced morbidity, and attenuated or stopped disease pro-gression, but no cure. Cessation of treatment ultimately will lead to relapse of the destructive inflammatory process. Traditional therapeu-tics include nonsteroidal antiinflammatory drugs (NSAID); immuno-suppressive drugs such as the so-called disease-modifying drugs metho-trexate (Chan and Cronstein 2002), sulfasalazine (Smedegard and Bjork 1995), and leflunomide (Fox et al. 1999); and glucocorticoids (Buttgereit et al. 2004). A prominent therapeutic strategy that stands for a more tar-geted therapy is the inhibition of proinflammatory cytokines using mon-oclonal antibodies or receptor–Ig fusion proteins (Fig. 1). The blocking of proinflammatory cytokines TNF-α (Scott and Kingsley 2006), IL-1 (Cohen 2004), and IL-6 (Nishimoto et al. 2004) that are abundantly ex-pressed at the site of inflammation has shown efficacy in RA. In particular, TNF-α antagonists represent a major therapeutic advancement in treatment of RA and other chronic inflammatory diseases such as ankylosing spondylitis and Crohn's disease, and highlight the potential of this approach (Nepom 2002; Panaccione et al. 2005).

Though the proposed mechanisms of action are different for these therapeutic strategies, their target is the same, namely an ongoing immune reaction. They affect parameters such as proliferation, cell activa-

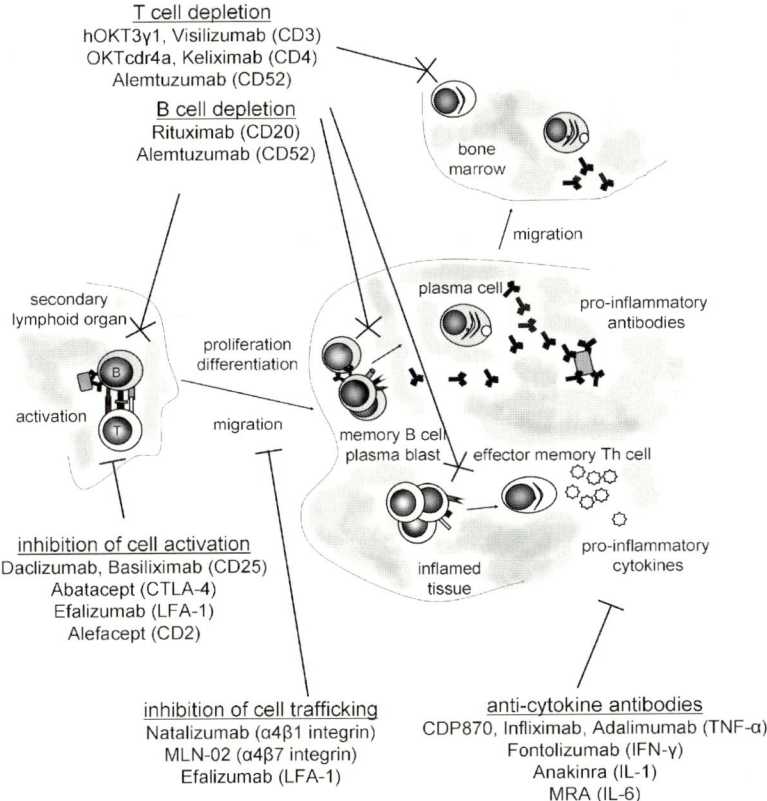

Fig. 1. Pathological mechanisms mediated by B and T cells are targets for therapeutic intervention. Selected biologicals and their target molecules are listed

tion, cytokine expression, and cell differentiation. Efficient systemic immunosuppression and immunomodulation are the bases of their efficacy, but also the reasons for their broad spectrum of adverse and side effects and impairment of immunocompetence. Their inability to cure may be due to either disease-driving mechanisms, which are independent of ongoing immune reactions, such as antigen-independent immune effector memory, as discussed above, or due to a resistance of chronic immune reactions to conventional immunosuppression. Alternative strategies of the future will aim at inhibition of migration and homing of proinflammatory cells, preventing their convention to reactivate and their presence in the target organ (Fig. 1). These targeted therapeutics will interfere with costimulatory requirements of advanced memory cells, e.g., ICOS, and they will aim at, as specifically as possible, the deletion of the cells driving disease, e.g., Th effector memory cells or autoreactive plasma cells (Nepom 2002; Panaccione et al. 2005).

5   Conclusion

The understanding of the mechanisms underlying chronic inflammation has improved over the last decades, and from it improved therapies have been developed. Still, those therapies do not provide a cure for chronic inflammatory diseases. This might be due to their insufficient interference with immunological memory. Proinflammatory immunological memory has been neglected so far as a prime candidate driving chronic inflammation. Therapeutic resolution of inflammation by suppression of ongoing pathogenic immune reactions may stop tissue destruction and associated immunopathology, and it may also result in the loss of survival niches for pathogenic memory cells resident in and dependent on the proinflammatory microenvironment of the inflamed tissue. However, resolution of inflammation will not affect memory cells that are located outside of the inflamed tissue, in particular long-lived pathogenic plasma cells and probably pathogenic effector memory T cells of the bone marrow as well (Di Rosa and Pabst 2005; Radbruch et al. 2006). The plasma cells will continue to provide pathogenic seed antibodies, a threshold and trigger of a relapse. It is a challenge for the development of future therapeutic strategies to target memory cells from the bone marrow, specifically the pathogenic ones, if possible.

References

Aarvak T, Chabaud M, Miossec P, Natvig JB (1999) IL-17 is produced by some proinflammatory Th1/Th0 cells but not by Th2 cells. J Immunol 162:1246–1251

Bernasconi NL, Traggiai E, Lanzavecchia A (2002) Maintenance of serological memory by polyclonal activation of human memory B cells. Science 298:2199–2202

Bernasconi NL, Onai N, Lanzavecchia A (2003) A role for Toll-like receptors in acquired immunity: up-regulation of TLR9 by BCR triggering in naive B cells and constitutive expression in memory B cells. Blood 101:4500–4504

Brennan FM, Foey AD, Feldmann M (2006) The importance of T cell interactions with macrophages in rheumatoid cytokine production. Curr Top Microbiol Immunol 305:177–194

Brewerton DA, Hart FD, Nicholls A, Caffrey M, James DC, Sturrock RD (1973) Ankylosing spondylitis and HL-A 27. Lancet 1:904–907

Brinkmann V, Kristofic C (1995) Regulation by corticosteroids of Th1 and Th2 cytokine production in human CD4$^+$ effector T cells generated from CD45RO$^-$ and CD45RO$^+$ subsets. J Immunol 155:3322–3328

Buttgereit F, Straub RH, Wehling M, Burmester GR (2004) Glucocorticoids in the treatment of rheumatic diseases: an update on the mechanisms of action. Arthritis Rheum 50:3408–3417

Calin A, Elswood J, Klouda PT (1989) Destructive arthritis, rheumatoid factor, and HLA-DR4. Susceptibility versus severity, a case-control study. Arthritis Rheum 32:1221–1225

Cambridge G, Leandro MJ, Edwards JC, Ehrenstein MR, Salden M, Bodman-Smith M, Webster AD (2003) Serologic changes following B lymphocyte depletion therapy for rheumatoid arthritis. Arthritis Rheum 48:2146–2154

Cassese G, Arce S, Hauser AE, Lehnert K, Moewes B, Mostarac M, Muehlinghaus G, Szyska M, Radbruch A, Manz RA (2003) Plasma cell survival is mediated by synergistic effects of cytokines and adhesion-dependent signals. J Immunol 171:1684–1690

Chan ES, Cronstein BN (2002) Molecular action of methotrexate in inflammatory diseases. Arthritis Res 4:266–273

Chan OT, Hannum LG, Haberman AM, Madaio MP, Shlomchik MJ (1999a) A novel mouse with B cells but lacking serum antibody reveals an antibody-independent role for B cells in murine lupus. J Exp Med 189:1639–1648

Chan OT, Madaio MP, Shlomchik MJ (1999b) B cells are required for lupus nephritis in the polygenic, Fas-intact MRL model of systemic autoimmunity. J Immunol 163:3592–3596

Chistiakov DA (2003) Thyroid-stimulating hormone receptor and its role in Graves' disease. Mol Genet Metab 80:377–388

Choy EH, Pitzalis C, Cauli A, Bijl JA, Schantz A, Woody J, Kingsley GH, Panayi GS (1996) Percentage of anti-CD4 monoclonal antibody-coated lymphocytes in the rheumatoid joint is associated with clinical improvement. Implications for the development of immunotherapeutic dosing regimens. Arthritis Rheum 39:52–56

Cohen SB (2004) The use of anakinra, an interleukin-1 receptor antagonist, in the treatment of rheumatoid arthritis (review). Rheum Dis Clin North Am 30:365–380, vii

Cohen SB, Emery P, Greenwald MW, Dougados M, Furie RA, Genovese MC, Keystone EC, Loveless JE, Burmester GR, Cravets MW, Hessey EW, Shaw T, Totoritis MC; REFLEX Trial Group (2006) Rituximab for rheumatoid arthritis refractory to antitumor necrosis factor therapy: results of a multicenter, randomized, double-blind, placebo-controlled, phase III trial evaluating primary efficacy and safety at twenty-four weeks. Arthritis Rheum 54:2793–2806

Cope AP (2002) Studies of T-cell activation in chronic inflammation. Arthritis Res 4(3):S197–S211

De Kleer IM, Brinkman DM, Ferster A, Abinun M, Quartier P, Van Der Net J, Ten Cate R, Wedderburn LR, Horneff G, Oppermann J, Zintl F, Foster HE, Prieur AM, Fasth A, Van Rossum MA, Kuis W, Wulffraat NM (2004) Autologous stem cell transplantation for refractory juvenile idiopathic arthritis: analysis of clinical effects, mortality, and transplant related morbidity. Ann Rheum Dis 63:1318–1326

Di Rosa F, Pabst R (2005) The bone marrow: a nest for migratory memory T cells. Trends Immunol 26:360–366

DiLorenzo TP, Serreze DV (2005) The good turned ugly: immunopathogenic basis for diabetogenic $CD8^+$ T cells in NOD mice. Immunol Rev 204:250–263

Dorner T, Hansen A (2004) Autoantibodies in normals—the value of predicting rheumatoid arthritis. Arthritis Res Ther 6:282–284

Drachman DB (1994) Myasthenia gravis. N Engl J Med 330:1797–1810

Edwards JC, Szczepanski L, Szechinski J, Filipowicz-Sosnowska A, Emery P, Close DR, Stevens RM, Shaw T (2004) Efficacy of B-cell-targeted therapy with rituximab in patients with rheumatoid arthritis. N Engl J Med 350:2572–2581

Ehinger M, Vestberg M, Johansson AC, Johannesson M, Svensson A, Holmdahl R (2001) Influence of CD4 or CD8 deficiency on collagen-induced arthritis. Immunology 103:291–300

Emery P, Fleischmann R, Filipowicz-Sosnowska A, Schechtman J, Szczepanski L, Kavanaugh A, Racewicz AJ, van Vollenhoven RF, Li NF, Agarwal S, Hessey EW, Shaw TM; DANCER Study Group (2006) The efficacy and safety of rituximab in patients with active rheumatoid arthritis despite methotrexate treatment: results of a phase IIB randomized, double-blind, placebo-controlled, dose-ranging trial. Arthritis Rheum 54:1390–1400

Falcone M, Lee J, Patstone G, Yeung B, Sarvetnick N (1998) B lymphocytes are crucial antigen-presenting cells in the pathogenic autoimmune response to GAD65 antigen in nonobese diabetic mice. J Immunol 161:1163–1168

Fox RI, Herrmann ML, Frangou CG, Wahl GM, Morris RE, Strand V, Kirschbaum BJ (1999) Mechanism of action for leflunomide in rheumatoid arthritis. Clin Immunol 93:198–208

Grayson JM, Harrington LE, Lanier JG, Wherry EJ, Ahmed R (2002) Differential sensitivity of naive and memory CD8$^+$ T cells to apoptosis in vivo. J Immunol 169:3760–3770

Horneff G, Burmester GR, Emmrich F, Kalden JR (1991) Treatment of rheumatoid arthritis with an anti-CD4 monoclonal antibody. Arthritis Rheum 34:129–140

Hoyer BF, Moser K, Hauser AE, Peddinghaus A, Voigt C, Eilat D, Radbruch A, Hiepe F, Manz RA (2004) Short-lived plasmablasts and long-lived plasma cells contribute to chronic humoral autoimmunity in NZB/W mice. J Exp Med 199:1577–1584

Iqbal N, Oliver JR, Wagner FH, Lazenby AS, Elson CO, Weaver CT (2002) T helper 1 and T helper 2 cells are pathogenic in an antigen-specific model of colitis. J Exp Med 195:71–84

Jayne D, Passweg J, Marmont A, et al. (2004) Autologous stem cell transplantation for systemic lupus erythematosus. Lupus 13:168–176

Kalia V, Sarkar S, Gourley TS, Rouse BT, Ahmed R (2006) Differentiation of memory B and T cells. Curr Opin Immunol 18:255–264

Keren DF, Kumar NB, Appelman HD (1987) Quantification of IgG-containing plasma cells as an adjunct to histopathology in distinguishing acute self-limited colitis from active idiopathic inflammatory bowel disease. Pathol Immunopathol Res 6:435–441

Klareskog L, Alfredsson L, Rantapaa-Dahlqvist S, Berglin E, Stolt P, Padyukov L (2004) What precedes development of rheumatoid arthritis? Ann Rheum Dis 63(2):ii28–ii31

Kohem CL, Brezinschek RI, Wisbey H, Tortorella C, Lipsky PE, Oppenheimer-Marks N (1996) Enrichment of differentiated CD45RBdim, CD27– memory T cells in the peripheral blood, synovial fluid, and synovial tissue of patients with rheumatoid arthritis. Arthritis Rheum 39:844–854

Kolls JK, Linden A (2004) Interleukin-17 family members and inflammation. Immunity 21:467–476

Korganow AS, Ji H, Mangialaio S, Duchatelle V, Pelanda R, Martin T, Degott C, Kikutani H, Rajewsky K, Pasquali JL, Benoist C, Mathis D (1999) From systemic T cell self-reactivity to organ-specific autoimmune disease via immunoglobulins. Immunity 10:451–461

Lafaille JJ, Keere FV, Hsu AL, Baron JL, Haas W, Raine CS, Tonegawa S (1997) Myelin basic protein-specific T helper 2 (Th2) cells cause experimental autoimmune encephalomyelitis in immunodeficient hosts rather than protect them from the disease. J Exp Med 186:307–312

Langrish CL, Chen Y, Blumenschein WM, Mattson J, Basham B, Sedgwick JD, McClanahan T, Kastelein RA, Cua DJ (2005) IL-23 drives a pathogenic T cell population that induces autoimmune inflammation. J Exp Med 201:233–240

Lanzavecchia A, Sallusto F (2005) Understanding the generation and function of memory T cell subsets. Curr Opin Immunol 17:326–332

Lau CM, Broughton C, Tabor AS, Akira S, Flavell RA, Mamula MJ, Christensen SR, Shlomchik MJ, Viglianti GA, Rifkin IR, Marshak-Rothstein A (2005) RNA-associated autoantigens activate B cells by combined B cell antigen receptor/Toll-like receptor 7 engagement. J Exp Med 202:1171–1177

Leadbetter EA, Rifkin IR, Hohlbaum AM, Beaudette BC, Shlomchik MJ, Marshak-Rothstein A (2002) Chromatin-IgG complexes activate B cells by dual engagement of IgM and Toll-like receptors. Nature 416:603–607

Leandro MJ, Cambridge G, Edwards JC, Ehrenstein MR, Isenberg DA (2005) B-cell depletion in the treatment of patients with systemic lupus erythematosus: a longitudinal analysis of 24 patients. Rheumatology (Oxford) 44:1542–1545

Lohning M, Richter A, Radbruch A (2002) Cytokine memory of T helper lymphocytes. Adv Immunol 80:115–181

Lohning M, Hutloff A, Kallinich T, Mages HW, Bonhagen K, Radbruch A, Hamelmann E, Kroczek RA (2003) Expression of ICOS in vivo defines CD4$^+$ effector T cells with high inflammatory potential and a strong bias for secretion of interleukin 10. J Exp Med 197:181–193

Machold KP, Stamm TA, Nell VP, Pflugbeil S, Aletaha D, Steiner G, Uffmann M, Smolen JS (2006) Very recent onset rheumatoid arthritis: clinical and serological patient characteristics associated with radiographic progression over the first years of disease. Rheumatology (Oxford) 46:342–349

Maffia P, Brewer JM, Gracie JA, Ianaro A, Leung BP, Mitchell PJ, Smith KM, McInnes IB, Garside P (2004) Inducing experimental arthritis and breaking self-tolerance to joint-specific antigens with trackable, ovalbumin-specific T cells. J Immunol 173:151–156

Miller JJ 3rd (1964) An autoradiographic study of plasma cell and lymphocyte survival in rat popliteal lymph nodes. J Immunol 92:673–681

Minges Wols HA, Underhill GH, Kansas GS, Witte PL (2002) The role of bone marrow-derived stromal cells in the maintenance of plasma cell longevity. J Immunol 169:4213–4221

Morita Y, Yamamura M, Kawashima M, Harada S, Tsuji K, Shibuya K, Maruyama K, Makino H (1998) Flow cytometric single-cell analysis of cytokine production by CD4$^+$ T cells in synovial tissue and peripheral blood from patients with rheumatoid arthritis. Arthritis Rheum 41:1669–1676

Muehlinghaus G, Cigliano L, Huehn S, Peddinghaus A, Leyendeckers H, Hauser AE, Hiepe F, Radbruch A, Arce S, Manz RA (2005) Regulation of CXCR3 and CXCR4 expression during terminal differentiation of memory B cells into plasma cells. Blood 105:3965–3971

Muraro PA, Douek DC, Packer A, Chung K, Guenaga FJ, Cassiani-Ingoni R, Campbell C, Memon S, Nagle JW, Hakim FT, Gress RE, McFarland HF, Burt RK, Martin R (2005) Thymic output generates a new and diverse TCR repertoire after autologous stem cell transplantation in multiple sclerosis patients. J Exp Med 201:805–816

Murphy CA, Langrish CL, Chen Y, Blumenschein W, McClanahan T, Kastelein RA, Sedgwick JD, Cua DJ (2003) Divergent pro- and antiinflammatory roles for IL-23 and IL-12 in joint autoimmune inflammation. J Exp Med 198:1951–1957

Nakajima C, Mukai T, Yamaguchi N, Morimoto Y, Park WR, Iwasaki M, Gao P, Ono S, Fujiwara H, Hamaoka T (2002) Induction of the chemokine receptor CXCR3 on TCR-stimulated T cells: dependence on the release from persistent TCR-triggering and requirement for IFN-gamma stimulation. Eur J Immunol 32:1792–1801

Nepom GT (2002) Therapy of autoimmune diseases: clinical trials and new biologics. Curr Opin Immunol 14:812–815

Nishimoto N, Yoshizaki K, Miyasaka N, Yamamoto K, Kawai S, Takeuchi T, Hashimoto J, Azuma J, Kishimoto T (2004) Treatment of rheumatoid arthritis with humanized anti-interleukin-6 receptor antibody: a multicenter, double-blind, placebo-controlled trial. Arthritis Rheum 50:1761–1769

Orme IM (1988) Characteristics and specificity of acquired immunologic memory to Mycobacterium tuberculosis infection. J Immunol 140:3589–3593

Panaccione R, Ferraz JG, Beck P (2005) Advances in medical therapy of inflammatory bowel disease. Curr Opin Pharmacol 5:566–572

Radbruch A, Muehlinghaus G, Luger EO, Inamine A, Smith KG, Dorner T, Hiepe F (2006) Competence and competition: the challenge of becoming a long-lived plasma cell. Nat Rev Immunol 6:741–750

Rantapaa-Dahlqvist S, de Jong BA, Berglin E, Hallmans G, Wadell G, Stenlund H, Sundin U, van Venrooij WJ (2003) Antibodies against cyclic citrullinated peptide and IgA rheumatoid factor predict the development of rheumatoid arthritis. Arthritis Rheum 48:2741–2749

Roosnek E, Lanzavecchia A (1991) Efficient and selective presentation of antigen-antibody complexes by rheumatoid factor B cells. J Exp Med 173:487–489

Rosen O, Thiel A, Massenkeil G, Hiepe F, Haupl T, Radtke H, Burmester GR, Gromnica-Ihle E, Radbruch A, Arnold R (2000) Autologous stem-cell transplantation in refractory autoimmune diseases after in vivo immunoablation and ex vivo depletion of mononuclear cells. Arthritis Res 2:327–336

Roth R, Nakamura T, Mamula MJ (1996) B7 costimulation and autoantigen specificity enable B cells to activate autoreactive T cells. J Immunol 157:2924–2931

Rotondi M, Lazzeri E, Romagnani P, Serio M (2003) Role for interferon-gamma inducible chemokines in endocrine autoimmunity: an expanding field. J Endocrinol Invest 26:177–180

Schroder AE, Greiner A, Seyfert C, Berek C (1996) Differentiation of B cells in the nonlymphoid tissue of the synovial membrane of patients with rheumatoid arthritis. Proc Natl Acad Sci USA 93:221–225

Scott DL, Kingsley GH (2006) Tumor necrosis factor inhibitors for rheumatoid arthritis. N Engl J Med 355:704–712

Slifka MK, Antia R, Whitmire JK, Ahmed R (1998) Humoral immunity due to long-lived plasma cells. Immunity 8:363–372

Smedegard G, Bjork J (1995) Sulphasalazine: mechanism of action in rheumatoid arthritis. Br J Rheumatol 34(2):7–15

Smith KG, Jones RB, Burns SM, Jayne DR (2006) Long-term comparison of rituximab treatment for refractory systemic lupus erythematosus and vasculitis: remission, relapse, and re-treatment. Arthritis Rheum 54:2970–2982

Suntharalingam G, Perry MR, Ward S, Brett SJ, Castello-Cortes A, Brunner MD, Panoskaltsis N (2006) Cytokine storm in a phase 1 trial of the anti-CD28 monoclonal antibody TGN1412. N Engl J Med 355:1018–1028

Taneja V, Taneja N, Paisansinsup T, Behrens M, Griffiths M, Luthra H, David CS (2002) CD4 and CD8 T cells in susceptibility/protection to collagen-induced arthritis in HLA-DQ8-transgenic mice: implications for rheumatoid arthritis. J Immunol 168:5867–5875

Thomas R, McIlraith M, Davis LS, Lipsky PE (1992) Rheumatoid synovium is enriched in CD45RBdim mature memory T cells that are potent helpers for B cell differentiation. Arthritis Rheum 35:1455–1465

Tsubaki T, Takegawa S, Hanamoto H, Arita N, Kamogawa J, Yamamoto H, Takubo N, Nakata S, Yamada K, Yamamoto S, Yoshie O, Nose M (2005) Accumulation of plasma cells expressing CXCR3 in the synovial sublining regions of early rheumatoid arthritis in association with production of Mig/CXCL9 by synovial fibroblasts. Clin Exp Immunol 141:363–371

Tyndall A, Saccardi R (2005) Haematopoietic stem cell transplantation in the treatment of severe autoimmune disease: results from phase I/II studies, prospective randomized trials and future directions. Clin Exp Immunol 141:1–9

Vencovsky J, Machacek S, Sedova L, Kafkova J, Gatterova J, Pesakova V, Ruzickova S (2003) Autoantibodies can be prognostic markers of an erosive disease in early rheumatoid arthritis. Ann Rheum Dis 62:427–430

Yang J, Zhu H, Murphy TL, Ouyang W, Murphy KM (2001) IL-18-stimulated GADD45 beta required in cytokine-induced, but not TCR-induced, IFN-gamma production. Nat Immunol 2:157–164

Yen D, Cheung J, Scheerens H, Poulet F, McClanahan T, McKenzie B, Kleinschek MA, Owyang A, Mattson J, Blumenschein W, Murphy E, Sathe M, Cua DJ, Kastelein RA, Rennick D (2006) IL-23 is essential for T cell-mediated colitis and promotes inflammation via IL-17 and IL-6. J Clin Invest 116:1310–1316

Ziolkowska M, Koc A, Luszczykiewicz G, Ksiezopolska-Pietrzak K, Klimczak E, Chwalinska-Sadowska H, Maslinski W (2000) High levels of IL-17 in rheumatoid arthritis patients: IL-15 triggers in vitro IL-17 production via cyclosporin A-sensitive mechanism. J Immunol 164:2832–2838

Ernst Schering Foundation Symposium Proceedings, Vol. 4, pp. 37–57
DOI 10.1007/2789_2007_038
© Springer-Verlag Berlin Heidelberg
Published Online: 15 June 2007

Post-transcriptional Regulators in Inflammation: Exploring New Avenues in Biological Therapeutics

V. Katsanou, M. Dimitriou, D.L. Kontoyiannis[(✉)]

BSRC "Alexander Fleming", Institute of Immunology, 34 Al. Fleming Str, 16672 Vari, Greece
email: *d.kontoyiannis@fleming.gr*

Abstract. The biosynthesis of inflammatory mediators relies on controlling the biogenesis and utilization of their corresponding messenger RNAs (mRNAs). These latter "utilization steps" encompass post-transcriptional mechanisms that gradually and variably impose a series of flexible-rate limiting controls to modify the abundance of an mRNA and the rate of its translation to protein in response to environmental signals. Mechanistically, post-transcriptional machines comprise networks of RNA binding proteins (RBPs), which recognize, passively or inducibly, secondary or tertiary ribonucleotide structures located on their target RNAs. The outcome of these interactions is the stringent control of mRNA maturation, localization, turnover and translation. It is conceivable that if these post-transcriptional interactions fail, they may perturb cellular responses to provide the impetus for chronic disease. Such is the case of the signal-responsive mechanisms affecting inflammatory mRNAs containing the AU-rich family of elements (AREs), which are recognized by a specific subset of RBPs. Intense research in this area has yielded important insight on the specific signals and mechanisms affecting the utilization of ARE-containing mRNAs. Here, we indicate briefly the inflammatory relevance of ARE-related mechanisms to highlight their importance in pathophysiology and their potential in the development of future biological therapies.

1   Introduction

The post-transcriptional regulation of inflammatory gene expression appears to have evolved as a homeostatic mechanism that defines the spatiotemporal pattern of an elicited immune response whilst preserving the balance between inflammation and tissue preservation. Current concepts favour that inflammatory signals determine the biosynthetic rate of cytokines, chemokines growth factors and small peptides by targeting specific ribonucleotide structures located in the corresponding messenger RNAs (mRNAs). Although in many instances the actual ribonucleotide structures responding to these signals remain unresolved, many may be inferred by a specific primary sequence composition whose binding has been validated by functional assays (mobility shift assays, genetic/biochemical/immunochemical RBP:RNA interaction screens, effects on reporter mRNA fate, etc.). Such is the case for the AU-rich family of elements (AREs) that are located in the untranslated regions (UTRs) of many inflammatory mRNAs and that are recognized by a specific subset of RNA-binding proteins (ARE-binding proteins; ARE-BPs).

2   Features of AU-Rich Elements

Evidence for the inducible post-transcriptional regulation of inflammatory mRNAs was provided during the late 1980s. It was found that cytokine mRNAs [such as those encoding tumour necrosis factors (TNFs), interleukins (ILs), interferons (IFNs) and colony-stimulating factors

(CSFs)] were labile and displayed accumulation profiles that were discordant to the levels of the proteins induced in stimulated innate cells. This effect was attributed to small AU-rich sequences present in the 3′ UTRs of these mRNAs, which could promote mRNA decay even when they were placed in the context of stable mRNAs (Shaw and Kamen 1986). Additional studies on cytokine mRNAs injected into Xenopus oocytes indicated that these elements could also block translation of cytokine mRNAs (Kruys et al. 1989). These early studies paved the way for a large amount of data collected over the last 15 years on what these sequences are and how they can modulate mRNA turnover and translation in response to numerous stimuli and in different cellular responses.

AREs are composed of a variable number of copies of the AUUUA or UUAUUUAUU nonamers and were originally classified into three separate functional subgroups based on their primary sequence (class I discontinuous nonamers; class II continuous/overlapping nonamers; class III undefined AU-rich structures) and the mode of mRNA degradation that they impose (Chen and Shyu 1995). In subsequent years and with the development of bioinformatics, large-scale computational approaches were performed to reveal an 8% distribution of AREs in mRNAs transcribed from human genes (Khabar 2005). These analyses indicated that ARE-containing transcripts are involved in transient and important cellular responses ranging from development and haematopoiesis to immune responses and cancer, rendering the AREs "pathophysiologically-relevant" RNA signatures. Based on the data assembled in the form of the ARE-containing mRNA database (ARED) (Bakheet et al. 2006), the ARE classification scheme was expanded to include five additional ARE subsets in class II AREs (clusters I–V relating to the number of nonamers).

Most of the biochemical studies performed to date highlight the importance of AREs in mediating the destabilization of eukaryotic transcripts. Although still under intense investigation, current concepts favour that AREs promote the shortening of the poly-A tail (deadenylation) and/or removal of the 5′ cap (decapping) (Xu et al. 1997; Wilusz et al. 2001). Degradation may then proceed through the recruitment of 5′–3′ exonucleases or through the sequestration of a complex of 3′–5′ exonucleases called the exosome (Chen and Shyu 1995; Mukherjee et al. 2002; Stoecklin et al. 2006). Despite the increasing knowledge of the biochemistry underlying ARE-mediated decay, the biochemical mechanisms mediating the potential of some AREs to block translation have not been analysed to the same extent. Instead such mechanisms have been inferred from functional studies (see also Sect. 3).

Notably, the heterogeneity amongst the ARE subsets indicates that their respective functions towards mRNA turnover and translation may vary amongst the different transcripts. For example, in bacterial lipopolysaccharide (LPS)-stimulated monocytes and IL-1-stimulated glioblastoma cell lines, representative mRNAs possessing class I AREs had slower decay rates than those with class II AREs (Frevel et al. 2003; Tebo et al. 2003). Current concepts favour that this heterogeneity may reflect the different interactions with ARE-binding proteins and signalling cascades. If that hypothesis holds true, then one should expect that the level of AREs' functional complexity rises multi-fold in the context of a signal-and-tissue specific response. Until the end of the 1990s, the limitations of biochemical and unicellular studies addressing ARE-mediated effects could not reveal the full potential of ARE-dependent modulation and their role in physio-pathological dynamics. With the turn of the century, the field was to be rejuvenated by the power of mammalian genetics and transgenic technologies.

2.1 Assessing the In Vivo Importance of AREs in Inflammation

The first indications that the post-transcriptional regulation of cytokine mRNAs can play important roles in immune physiology came from studies correlating abnormal patterns of TNF expression with inflammatory disease. TNF plays a central role in various immune and inflammatory phenomena by eliciting differential signals in target cells ranging from cellular activation and proliferation to cytotoxicity and apoptosis. Biological anti-TNF therapies in chronic inflammatory diseases have been very successful in the clinic (Feldmann and Maini 2001), but are not without side-effects towards infection and autoimmunity, necessitating the discovery of alternative approaches. Early *in vitro* works have indicated that the presence of a conserved AU-rich element in the 3′ UTR of the TNF mRNA (now classified as a prototypical class II ARE) could affect the inducible expression of this molecule in innate cells (Caput et al. 1986). Most intriguingly, the replacement of this 3′ UTR with that from the β-globin mRNA was sufficient to drive TNF overexpression in transgenic mice supporting the development of numerous pathologies (depending on the promoters used to drive expression of these transgenes) including arthritis and systemic and CNS inflammation (Douni et al. 1995; Kollias et al. 2002). At the same time, genetic analysis of lupus-prone mice indicated that a spontaneous dinucleotide disruption of the TNF 3′ ARE reduced the levels of TNF biosynthesis, supporting the development of autoimmune disease (Jacob and Tashman 1993); however, gene targeting in embryonic stem (ES) cells was meant to provide the definitive proof of the TNF3′ ARE function. The obligatory or conditional targeted deletion of this 69-bp element from the mouse TNF locus resulted in severe polyarthritic and inflammatory bowel disease (IBD) phenotypes with resemblance to the human conditions of Crohn's disease and rheumatoid arthritis (Kontoyiannis et al. 1999, 2001). In the absence of the ARE, the inducible production of TNF from mouse macrophages and lymphocytes was excessively prolonged, supporting a continuous state of innate activation as well as hypersensitivity to inflammatory agonists (Kontoyiannis et al. 1999, 2001, 2002). In addition, this small deletion was sufficient to drive the ectopic expression of TNF in cells that do not normally produce this cytokine (e.g. synovial fibroblasts), indicating that the AREs modulate both temporal and spatial parameters of mRNA expression (Kontoyiannis et al. 1999). In molecular terms, these phenomena were attributed to the increased stability of the TNF mRNA and the absence of translational silencing mechanisms (Kontoyiannis et al. 1999, 2001, 2002).

One important point that these studies revealed was that the AREs can respond both to immune-activating and immune-suppressive signals. For example, the absence of the TNF3′ ARE rendered this cytokine partially or totally unresponsive to the anti-inflammatory effects of corticosteroids, nonsteroidal anti-inflammatory drugs (NSAIDs) and natural antagonists such as IL-10 (Kontoyiannis et al. 1999, 2001). The inability of IL-10 to modulate TNF biosynthesis due to the absence of TNF3′ ARE appears as a key deterministic parameter for the development of inflammatory disease, as was exemplified in the case of TNF-induced IBD (Kontoyiannis et al. 2002). Whether IL-10 targets the ARE-dependent modulation of TNF mRNA translation, stability or both is still a matter of debate, although signal- and species-specific variations may be responsible for these discrepancies. It is conceivable that other anti-inflammatory cues may also be affected as has been previously suggested for the IL-4 and IL-13 mediated suppression of TNF biosynthesis (Mijatovic et al. 1997).

The importance of class II AREs in the maintenance of homeostasis was also indicated in transgenic studies for the granulocyte-macrophage colony-stimulating factor (GM-CSF) mRNA (Houzet et al. 2001). In this case the early developmental expression of GM-CSF mRNA was permissive only when its ARE was deleted. This deletion had severe consequences for myelopoiesis manifested by the abnormal accumulation of myeloid progenitors, the increased proliferation of granulocytes and macrophages, and embryonic lethality, presumably due to an increase in GM-CSF mRNA stability and/or translation.

These results, however, should be cautiously considered and should not be generalized for all mRNAs containing AREs. This was exemplified in a third series of transgenic systems examining the effects of the c-*myc* 3' UTR that possesses a different ARE signature from those found on the TNF and GM-CSF mRNAs. Despite numerous previous in vitro studies pointing towards the important role of c-*myc* ARE in the modulation of c-*myc* mRNA stability, its deletion from the corresponding c-*myc* encoding transgenes had nominal effects in their expression and mouse physiology (Langa et al. 2001). Thus, and as proposed earlier, the heterogeneity amongst different AREs may in fact indicate different ARE-mediated effects that can only be revealed in an in vivo context, as it occurs in the transgenic systems of ARE deletion described above.

As is clear from the studies on TNF mRNA in inflammation, AREs appear to respond to numerous signals to maintain the homoeostasis of a given response. Thus, the elucidation of "ARE signalosomes" is of high clinical and pharmacological importance; it reveals putative targets for pathology. In the following section we will indicate briefly the importance of specific signal transduction pathways targeting the AREs in inflammation that have been validated in transgenic systems.

2.2   Inflammatory ARE Signalosomes

Most of the current knowledge on signals affecting the post-transcriptional regulation of immune mRNAs is derived from studies on innate effector cells (e.g. macrophages). Apart from their importance as cellular mediators of inflammation, innate cells are excellent systems to study inflammatory gene expression due to their capacity to readily produce cytokines, chemokines and acute phase proteins in response to defined infectious activators and inflammatory signals. As the intricacies of Toll-like receptors (TLRs) and cytokine receptors [tumour necrosis factor receptors (TNFRs), IL-1 receptor (IL-1R) and IFN receptors (IFNRs)] are being unveiled, it is becoming clear that their signals target post-transcriptional modules. For example, the engagement of the classical TLR4 pathway on macrophages triggers positive changes in stability and the translation of TNF, IL-1, IL-3, IL-6, IL-8 and cyclo-oxygenase-2 (COX-2) mRNAs (Kracht and Saklatvala 2002).

In 1994 a class of pyridinyl imidazole compounds was identified that blocked these post-transcriptional changes, through binding to members of the serine/threonine family of p38 stress-activated protein kinases (kinases) (Lee and Young 1996). Through the use of such small molecule inhibitors and transgenic systems, the intense research that followed revealed that the p38α/β isoforms modulate the stability and the translation of cytokine mRNAs that contain AREs. This effect is primarily mediated through the p38-mediated activation of the downstream mitogen-activated protein kinase activated protein kinase 2 (MAPKAPK-2 or MK2) and to a lesser extent by MAPKAPK-3 (MK3) that target ARE-binding proteins (Gaestel 2006; see also Sect. 3). Mutant mice with a deficiency in MK2 are resistant to models of endotoxemia and collagen-induced arthritis, whereas they remain sensitive to intracellular pathogens, reciprocating states of TNF/TNFR deficiency (Kotlyarov et al. 1999; Lehner et al. 2002; Hegen et al. 2006). These effects have been partially attributed the lack of MK2 modulation on the ARE-dependent translation/stabilization of cytokine mRNAs such as those encoding TNF and IL-6 (Gaestel 2006; Neininger et al. 2002). The wealth of data on the p38/MK2 axis towards cytokine biosynthesis provided solid support for the development of new biological therapies targeting these molecules in inflammatory disease with promising effects for rheumatoid arthritis, IBDs and lung inflammation (Saklatvala 2004; Peifer et al. 2006; Adcock et al. 2006). However, the p38/MK2 cascade appears to modulate a pleiotropy of cellular signals extending beyond their effects on cytokine biosynthesis (Gaestel 2006; Ashwell 2006). In addition they may cross-react with numerous additional cascades [such as the nuclear factor κB (NFκB)-related kinases and other MAPKs and stress-activated protein kinases (SAPKs); Karin 2005] and thus their respective blockade may lack the necessary "kinome" selectivity to target exclusively an anti-inflammatory effect, particularly in the case of chronic inflammation. Such an example has been provided in a genetic mouse model of Crohn's disease, where MK2 deficiency resulted in exacerbated inflammation in the intestinal mucosa, attributed to the lack of p38-mediated apoptotic control of infiltrating cells (Kontoyiannis et al. 2002).

Additional TLR-associated signals converging to AREs have been described and include c-Jun N-terminal kinase (JNK) isoforms, the MAP3 kinase Tpl2/Cot and the extracellular signal-regulated kinase 1/2 (ERK1/2) MAPK revealing additional signal-induced ARE-mediated effects such as nucleocytoplasmic mRNA transport (Kontoyiannis et al. 1999, 2001; Dumitru et al. 2000). Furthermore, ARE-related signalling cross-talks emanating from the concomitant engagement of inflammatory and anti- or co-inflammatory receptors [TLR to MAPK modules versus IL-10/IFNs to Janus kinase (JAK)/signal transducer and activator of transcription (STAT)/suppressors of cytokine signalling (SOCS) modules] have been described; whether these effects are directly targeting specific ARE-mediated processes or are interfering with the p38/MK pathway is currently unclear, although evidence for the latter has been provided in the case of IL-10 associated signals (Kontoyiannis et al. 2001; Rajasingh et al. 2006).

Overall the clinical exploitation of these signalling cascades provides the first line of evidence for the importance of post-transcriptional modules as putative therapeutic targets. To identify more targets of increased specificity, current research is focussing on the terminal acceptors of inflammatory signals, i.e. the RNA binding proteins that modulate mRNA turnover and translation.

3   Determinants of Fate: ARE-BPs

The RBP genes constitute of one of the largest gene families conserved across species, which may reflect the pleiotropy of their functions. It appears, however, that the determination of mRNA fate is the collective sum of numerous RBPs assembled in ribonucleoprotein particles (RNPs). The dynamics between RBPs and RNAs in RNPs are complex and difficult to monitor in the context of complex cellular response, e.g. the inflammatory response; however, they can be inferred by the effects of individual RBP components on their mRNA targets as reflected in the paradigm of ARE-dependent modulation. Numerous ARE-binding proteins (ARE-BPs) have been identified to date (Barreau et al. 2006); however, a few have been implicated in the control of ARE-containing mRNAs. Most of them have been associated with negative effects on mRNA fate, i.e. destabilization or translational silencing, whereas only one family—the Elavl/Hu—has been described as a positive regulator. These proteins contain different protein motifs through which they recognize RNA structures, suggesting that the AREs are "modular" in nature and consist of different binding sites. In the following sections we will focus on those ARE-BPs that have a proven involvement in inflammatory reactions, as has been suggested in studies using transgenic mammals.

3.1   Tristetraprolin Family

The tristetraprolin (TTP) family of CCCH tandem zinc-finger proteins is composed of four known members in mammals, three of which are highly conserved in humans and rodents (Zfp36/TTP, Zfp36L1/BRF1, Zfp36L2/BRF1). All members have the restricted capacity to recognize class II AREs and promote deadenylation-dependent destabilization of the transcripts they bind (Blackshear 2002). The prototype member of this family, TTP, is now known to affect the turnover of specific mRNA subsets. The generation of TTP-deficient mice, however, revealed that the functions of this molecule are primarily related to the haematopoietic and myeloid responses. These mice develop a systemic inflammatory syndrome with severe polyarticular arthritis and myeloid hyperplasia. The syndrome seemed to be due predominantly to excess tumour necrosis factor-alpha (TNF-alpha) and GM-CSF, resulting from the increased stability of the TNF-alpha and GM-CSF mRNAs (Carrick et al. 2004). The molecular specifics of TTP functioning have been highlighted recently (Gaestel 2006). TTP is phosphorylated by MK2 in LPS-stimulated macrophages; this phosphorylation event appears to increase TTP protein stability and provide anchorage sites for binding to 14-3-3 proteins. This interaction prohibits the sequestration of TTP to its targets, thus inhibiting its destabilizing effect. Consequently the p38/MK2-dependent interaction of TTP to 14-3-3 is alleviated, presumably via protein phosphatases such as protein phosphatase 2A (PP2A), and TTP is activated to suppress the potentially harmful production of inflammatory mediators (Sun et al. 2006). In addition, the TTP mRNA and protein appear to be heavily regulated at the post-transcriptional (even by itself) and post-translational levels, as in the case of many of its target mRNAs (Brook et al. 2006; Hitti et al. 2006). These findings render TTP as the first RNA binding protein with a specific relevance to inflammatory responses and suggest that strategies aiming towards the augmentation of its functions (either by affecting its phosphorylation status or increasing its abundance) can have a clear clinical benefit in inflammatory conditions such as rheumatoid arthritis.

A similar mode of function has been recently described for the second family member, Zfp36L1/BRF1, that responds to protein kinase B (PKB) signals (Benjamin et al. 2006). Unfortunately, mice deficient for this molecule, die at early embryonic stages, thus prohibiting the assessment of the molecules' functions in inflammation (Stumpo et al. 2004; Ramos et al. 2004). However, it is highly likely that these proteins play similar roles—either in other cellular compartments (e.g. lymphocytes) or in response to additional inflammatory signalling cascades—which will be revealed in the future.

3.2   TIA-1/TIAR

TIA-1 and TIAR are closely related members of the RNA recognition motif (RRM) family of RNA-binding proteins binding to numerous mRNAs containing a U-rich motif. Both proteins inhibit the translation of TNF transcripts in macrophages. TIA-1 deficient mice are phenotypically normal, but in one specific genetic background they display mild symptoms of arthritis (Phillips et al. 2004; Piecyk et al. 2000). These mice also appear very sensitive to mouse models of endotoxemia (Piecyk et al. 2000). TIA-1 deficient macrophages overproduce TNF-alpha protein and the percentage of TNF transcripts found in polysomes is significantly increased, suggesting that TIA-1 functions as a translational silencer (Piecyk et al. 2000).

The mechanism of TIA-1 functions has been revealed in vitro, using cellular systems of oxidative stress-induced phosphorylation of eukaryotic initiation factor 2α (eIF2α), prohibiting the initiation of protein synthesis. Under these conditions, TIA-1 assembles with components of translation-initiation machinery which is directed at discrete cytoplasmic foci known as stress granules (SGs) (Anderson and Kedersha 2006). Stress granules are also rich in RNP complexes and thus are regarded as "decision making" sites where mRNAs are stalled prior to their destruction or translation. The recent demonstration that phosphorylated TTP is excluded from SGs whereas its non-phosphorylated form is present conforms to this notion and suggests that translational inhibition is indirectly linked to destabilization (Stoecklin and Anderson 2006).

Although these molecular events have not been clearly demonstrated in innate cells, due to the rapidity of their response, it is highly likely that they occur in a similar fashion. This is further exemplified in mice rendered deficient for both TIA-1 and TTP, where they develop a much-exacerbated form of arthritis compared the ones observed in either singly deficient mouse (Phillips et al. 2004). However, this result was accompanied with the puzzling observation that TTP/TIA-1 double-deficient macrophages produced very low amounts of TNF, whereas the major source of TNF overexpression was restricted to granulocytes. This points towards the existence of additional "silencer" molecules functioning in macrophages.

It is currently unclear whether a strategy aimed at augmenting TIA-1 functions could have a beneficial effect as an anti-inflammatory strategy; however, if TIA-1 is a requirement for "stalling" mRNAs in SGs and allows for their indirect tethering towards destabilization, then such an approach may have a wider application versus strategies affecting TTP.

3.3 AUF1

Historically, AUF was the first ARE-binding protein cloned, but most of the knowledge on this molecule does not directly relate to inflammation. AUF1 also belongs to the family of RRM-containing RBPs and exists as four different isoforms, p37, p40, p42 and p45, which result from differential splicing. AUF1 binds to numerous cytokine and growth-factor mRNAs in vitro, although the full spectrum of its affinities have not been determined. Interestingly both destabilizing and stabilizing roles for AUF1 have been suggested from the results of unicellular overexpression experiments (Wilson and Brewer 1999). The multiple isoforms of AUF1, however, may have different roles in different cell types and have not been individually analysed. Similarly to TTP, AUF1 is phosphorylated in vivo (Wilson et al. 2003), indicating a more prominent response to proliferating and stress signals. A very recent report describing the generation of an AUF1-deficient mouse revealed the potential implication of this ARE-BP also in the modulation of inflammatory cascades. AUF1-deficient mice show a mild growth-retardation phenotype but also appear relatively more sensitive to endotoxemia than wild-type controls (Lu et al. 2006). Although this effect is partially attributed to increases in TNF and IL-1β mRNA stability in macrophages, there is no clear cellular or molecular evidence that AUF1 acts in an anti-inflammatory fashion. Still, these findings render AUF1 as putative target for inflammatory disorders that need to be examined more thoroughly in the future.

3.4 Elavl1/HuR

HuR is the prototypical member of the *Elavl/Hu* family of RNA-binding proteins named after the lethal phenotypes of their homologue in *Drosophila* (embryonic lethal abnormal vision) and their appearance as specific tumour antigens in individuals with paraneoplastic neurological disorders (Hu antigens). In mammals the family is composed of the ubiquitously expressed HuR (HuA or Elavl1) and the neuronal-specific HuB, HuC and HuD. HuR has a prototypical RBP structure that includes two N-terminal RRMs with high affinity for a U-rich sequence (HuR binding motif, HBM), followed by a nucleocytoplasmic shuttling sequence and a C-terminal RRM recognizing the poly-A tail (Fan and Steitz 1998; Fan and Steitz 1998; Lopez de Silanes et al. 2004). Although predominantly nuclear, HuR shuttles between the nucleus and the cytoplasm acting as an RNA adaptor. Numerous studies have indicated that the cytoplasmic HuR can stabilize specific mRNAs (Brennan and Steitz 2001). However, the constitutive and high expression of HuR and the wide distribution of HBM among numerous ARE/non-ARE-containing mRNAs indicate that HuR recognition may not be very discriminative, hence the mechanisms involved in inducing the specificity of its functions remain elusive. With respect to inflammation, studies on macrophage cell lines suggested that innate sensitizers increase the cytoplasmic binding of HuR to cytokine mRNAs supporting their stabilization (Brennan and Steitz 2001; Dean et al. 2004). Furthermore, genetic approaches have identified mouse strains with mutations in the HBM of inflammatory mRNAs that correlate with the development of autoimmunity (Di Marco et al. 2001). These observations suggest that the overt upregulation of HuR could support the hyper-activation of inflammatory mediators to drive ensuing inflammation. However, the search for HuR's role in inflammation has been obstructed by its predictive involvement in central developmental processes (Levadoux-Martin et al. 2003), which have been recently confirmed in HuR-deficient mice (V. Katsanou and D.L. Kontoyiannis, unpublished).

The positive role of HuR towards cytokine biosynthesis was recently challenged through in vivo systems of tetracycline-inducible and macrophage-specific overexpression in the mouse (Katsanou et al. 2005). These mice displayed reduced in vivo inflammatory responses in modelled endotoxemia and were resistant in modelled hepatitis. The anti-inflammatory effect of the transgenic HuR correlated with the reduced production of a specific set of inflammatory mediators, indicating that in vivo, HuR acts in a discriminative fashion. HuR was found to associate directly with TNF, COX-2 and transforming growth factor beta 1 (TGFβ1) mRNAs and indirectly with the IL-1β mRNA, consequently blocking the biosynthesis of the corresponding proteins in stimulated transgenic macrophages. The most surprising finding was that HuR overexpression reduced the translation of these inflammatory mRNAs, although it increased the stability of class II mRNAs (such as TNF and

COX-2 AREs), as has been previously suggested. The genetic elimination of TTP and TIA-1 in the context of HuR overexpression revealed a synergy between the corresponding functions of these RBPs towards the modulation of TNF mRNA translation; HuR required the functions of TIA-1 to inhibit the translation of TNF mRNA and this effect occurred even in the absence of TTP deficiency. By combining the current data on HuR, TTP and TIA-1, these studies postulate a functional hierarchy towards the modulation of mRNAs bearing class II AREs, where HuR is tethering such mRNAs towards TIA-1-mediated translational inhibition, which in turn tethers towards destabilization by TTP. This is also compatible with the inclusion of all three RBPs in stress granules and the fact that the HBM is distinct from the binding sites of other RBPs (Keene and Tenenbaum 2002; Lopez de Silanes et al. 2005).

The molecular details and the widespread representation for this "consequential tethering model" remain to be determined. Clues as to its necessity, however, are starting to come forth. The data provided from HuR transgenic studies indicate that the functions of this molecule are not definite but may be governed by the modular constitution of the ARE niche (i.e. the HBM with or without ARE of different class or cluster) in each independent mRNA species. For example, the TNF and COX-2 mRNAs that contain an HBM next to a class II- cluster III ARE and respond similarly to HuR in stimulated macrophages (increased stability, reduced translation) are targets for TTP and TIA-1. On the other hand, the TGFβ1 mRNA contains an HBM but does not contain a prototypical ARE; HuR overexpression reduces its translation and is not a target for TTP, although it is unknown whether or not it binds to TIA-1/TIA-R. This points towards a role for HuR in organizing the mRNAs in "functional clusters" required for an elicited response. This, in fact, has been proposed by Keene and Tenenbaum (2002) based on en masse, RBP-coupled RNA immunoprecipitation studies where it was demonstrated that Hu-containing RNPs contain functionally related mRNAs. We postulate that, at least in macrophages, HuR acts as a co-ordinator of downstream RBP associations that will be governed by the quantity and the intrinsic properties of a given mRNA subset, as well as the activation of specific RBPs in response to an external stimulus. Although this property of HuR remains to be validated in systems of HuR deficiency, it reveals the increased potential of future therapeutic strategies aiming at the overexpression of this molecule in inflammation.

4   Concluding Remarks

This brief review aims to suggest to the prospective reader that post-transcriptional signalosomes and RBPs identify connections between genes and disease, and thus their analysis can provide better diagnostics and therapeutics. For the paradigm of inflammation, we postulate that targeting selective tissue-specific RNA:RBP associations in disease will provide better means for therapeutic intervention since a specific collection of functionally related pathogenic-effector products will be targeted instead of (1) a select few (e.g. antibodies to selected inflammatory mediators) that can have marginal effects on disease progression or (2) non-specifically too many (e.g. chemical inhibitors of receptors or intracellular signals affecting a wide spectrum of transcriptional, post-transcriptional and post-translational mechanisms) that current therapeutic schemes are focussed upon. The development of such therapeutic schemes, however, will have to rely on the outcome of the studies analysing RBPs in a tissue-specific context. For example, even though the analyses of ARE-mediated mechanisms in inflammation have made tremendous strides over the last few years, they is still quite limited. First, the mechanics of ARE-BP functions remain unresolved, especially in light of new data that indicate the interplay of these proteins with modulating micro-RNA subsets (Bhattacharyya et al. 2006; Jing et al. 2005). Second, and concerning inflammation, most of the current knowledge is derived from the analysis of innate cells in response to a limited number of signals. The molecular and cellular attributes of ARE-dependent modulation in other inflammatory effectors (i.e. lymphocytes, endothelia, etc.) and targets (e.g. epithelia, neurons, etc.) are largely unknown. It is almost certain, however, that the coupling conditional transgenic technologies to molecular and functional genomics' platforms will reveal the pathophysiological role for RBPs and signalling cascades in support of a novel class of biological therapeutics targeting post-transcriptional processes.

Acknowledgements. The authors wish to thank George Kollias and members of his lab for the collaborative studies on the TNF ARE and its role in immune disease. This work was supported by funding under the Sixth Research Framework Programme of the European Union, Project MUGEN (MUGEN LSHB-CT-2005-005203) and the Hellenic Secretariat for Research and Technology grants PENED-2003-3EΔ770 and PENED-2003-3EΔ264

References

Adcock IM, Chung KF, Caramori G, Ito K (2006) Kinase inhibitors and airway inflammation. Eur J Pharmacol 533:118–132

Anderson P, Kedersha N (2006) RNA granules. J Cell Biol 172:803–808

Ashwell JD (2006) The many paths to p38 mitogen-activated protein kinase activation in the immune system. Nat Rev Immunol 6:532–540

Bakheet T, Williams BR, Khabar KS (2006) ARED 3: the large and diverse AU-rich transcriptome. Nucleic Acids Res 34:D111–D114

Barreau C, Paillard L, Osborne HB (2006) AU-rich elements and associated factors: are there unifying principles? Nucleic Acids Res 33:7138–7150

Benjamin D, Schmidlin M, Min L, Gross B, Moroni C (2006) BRF1 protein turnover and mRNA decay activity are regulated by protein kinase B at the same phosphorylation sites. Mol Cell Biol 26:9497–9507

Bhattacharyya SN, Habermacher R, Martine U, Closs EI, Filipowicz W (2006) Relief of microRNA-mediated translational repression in human cells subjected to stress. Cell 125:1111–1124

Blackshear PJ (2002) Tristetraprolin and other CCCH tandem zinc-finger proteins in the regulation of mRNA turnover. Biochem Soc Trans 30:945–952

Brennan CM, Steitz JA (2001) HuR and mRNA stability. Cell Mol Life Sci 58:266–277

Brook M, Tchen CR, Santalucia T, McIlrath J, Arthur JS, Saklatvala J, Clark AR (2006) Posttranslational regulation of tristetraprolin subcellular localization and protein stability by p38 mitogen-activated protein kinase and extracellular signal-regulated kinase pathways. Mol Cell Biol 26:2408–2418

Caput D, Beutler B, Hartog K, Thayer R, Brown-Shimer S, Cerami A (1986) Identification of a common nucleotide sequence in the 3′-untranslated region of mRNA molecules specifying inflammatory mediators. Proc Natl Acad Sci USA 83:1670–1674

Carrick DM, Lai WS, Blackshear PJ (2004) The tandem CCCH zinc finger protein tristetraprolin and its relevance to cytokine mRNA turnover and arthritis. Arthritis Res Ther 6:248–264

Chen CY, Shyu AB (1995) AU-rich elements: characterization and importance in mRNA degradation. Trends Biochem Sci 20:465–470

Dean JL, Sully G, Clark AR, Saklatvala J (2004) The involvement of AU-rich element-binding proteins in p38 mitogen-activated protein kinase pathway-mediated mRNA stabilisation. Cell Signal 16:1113–1121

Di Marco S, Hel Z, Lachance C, Furneaux H, Radzioch D (2001) Polymorphism in the 3′-untranslated region of TNFalpha mRNA impairs binding of the post-transcriptional regulatory protein HuR to TNFalpha mRNA. Nucleic Acids Res 29:863–871

Douni E, Akassoglou K, Alexopoulou L, Georgopoulos S, Haralambous S, Hill S, Kassiotis G, Kontoyiannis D, Pasparakis M, Plows D, Probert L, Kollias G (1995) Transgenic and knockout analyses of the role of TNF in immune regulation and disease pathogenesis. J Inflamm 47:27–38

Dumitru CD, Ceci JD, Tsatsanis C, Kontoyiannis D, Stamatakis K, Lin JH, Patriotis C, Jenkins NA, Copeland NG, Kollias G, Tsichlis PN (2000) TNF-alpha induction by LPS is regulated posttranscriptionally via a Tpl2/ERK-dependent pathway. Cell 103:1071–1083

Fan XC, Steitz JA (1998) HNS, a nuclear-cytoplasmic shuttling sequence in HuR. Proc Natl Acad Sci USA 95:15293–15298

Fan XC, Steitz JA (1998) Overexpression of HuR, a nuclear-cytoplasmic shuttling protein, increases the in vivo stability of ARE-containing mRNAs. EMBO J 17:3448–3460

Feldmann M, Maini RN (2001) Anti-TNF alpha therapy of rheumatoid arthritis: what have we learned? Annu Rev Immunol 19:163–196

Frevel MA, Bakheet T, Silva AM, Hissong JG, Khabar KS, Williams BR (2003) p38 Mitogen-activated protein kinase-dependent and -independent signaling of mRNA stability of AU-rich element-containing transcripts. Mol Cell Biol 23:425–436

Gaestel M (2006) MAPKAP kinases—MKs—two's company, three's a crowd. Nat Rev Mol Cell Biol 7:120–130

Hegen M, Gaestel M, Nickerson-Nutter CL, Lin LL, Telliez JB (2006) MAP-KAP kinase 2-deficient mice are resistant to collagen-induced arthritis. J Immunol 177:1913–1917

Hitti E, Iakovleva T, Brook M, Deppenmeier S, Gruber AD, Radzioch D, Clark AR, Blackshear PJ, Kotlyarov A, Gaestel M (2006) Mitogen-activated protein kinase-activated protein kinase 2 regulates tumor necrosis factor mRNA stability and translation mainly by altering tristetraprolin expression, stability, and binding to adenine/uridine-rich element. Mol Cell Biol 26:2399–2407

Houzet L, Morello D, Defrance P, Mercier P, Huez G, Kruys V (2001) Regulated control by granulocyte-macrophage colony-stimulating factor AU-rich element during mouse embryogenesis. Blood 98:1281–1288

Jacob CO, Tashman NB (1993) Disruption in the AU motif of the mouse TNF-alpha 3′ UTR correlates with reduced TNF production by macrophages in vitro. Nucleic Acids Res 21:2761–2766

Jing Q, Huang S, Guth S, Zarubin T, Motoyama A, Chen J, Di PF, Lin SC, Gram H, Han J (2005) Involvement of microRNA in AU-rich element-mediated mRNA instability. Cell 120:623–634

Karin M (2005) Inflammation-activated protein kinases as targets for drug development. Proc Am Thorac Soc 2:386–390

Katsanou V, Papadaki O, Milatos S, Blackshear PJ, Anderson P, Kollias G, Kontoyiannis DL (2005) HuR as a negative posttranscriptional modulator in inflammation. Mol Cell 19:777–789

Keene JD, Tenenbaum SA (2002) Eukaryotic mRNPs may represent posttranscriptional operons. Mol Cell 9:1161–1167

Khabar KS (2005) The AU-rich transcriptome: more than interferons and cytokines, and its role in disease. J Interferon Cytokine Res 25:1–10

Kollias G, Kontoyiannis D, Douni E, Kassiotis G (2002) The role of TNF/TNFR in organ-specific and systemic autoimmunity: implications for the design of optimized "anti-TNF" therapies. Curr Dir Autoimmun 5:30–50

Kontoyiannis D, Pasparakis M, Pizarro TT, Cominelli F, Kollias G (1999) Impaired on/off regulation of TNF biosynthesis in mice lacking TNF AU-rich elements: implications for joint and gut-associated immunopathologies. Immunity 10:387–398

Kontoyiannis D, Kotlyarov A, Carballo E, Alexopoulou L, Blackshear PJ, Gaestel M, Davis R, Flavell R, Kollias G (2001) Interleukin-10 targets p38 MAPK to modulate ARE-dependent TNF mRNA translation and limit intestinal pathology. EMBO J 20:3760–3770

Kontoyiannis D, Boulougouris G, Manoloukos M, Armaka M, Apostolaki M, Pizarro T, Kotlyarov A, Forster I, Flavell R, Gaestel M, Tsichlis P, Cominelli F, Kollias G (2002) Genetic dissection of the cellular pathways and signaling mechanisms in modeled tumor necrosis factor-induced Crohn's-like inflammatory bowel disease. J Exp Med 196:1563–1574

Kotlyarov A, Neininger A, Schubert C, Eckert R, Birchmeier C, Volk HD, Gaestel M (1999) MAPKAP kinase 2 is essential for LPS-induced TNF-alpha biosynthesis. Nat Cell Biol 1:94–97

Kracht M, Saklatvala J (2002) Transcriptional and post-transcriptional control of gene expression in inflammation. Cytokine 20:91–106

Kruys V, Marinx O, Shaw G, Deschamps J, Huez G (1989) Translational blockade imposed by cytokine-derived UA-rich sequences. Science 245:852–855

Langa F, Lafon I, Vandormael-Pournin S, Vidaud M, Babinet C, Morello D (2001) Healthy mice with an altered c-myc gene: role of the 3′ untranslated region revisited. Oncogene 20:4344–4353

Lee JC, Young PR (1996) Role of CSB/p38/RK stress response kinase in LPS and cytokine signaling mechanisms. J Leukoc Biol 59:152–157

Lehner MD, Schwoebael F, Kotlyarov A, Leist M, Gaestel M, Hartung T (2002) Mitogen-activated protein kinase-activated protein kinase 2-deficient mice show increased susceptibility to Listeria monocytogenes infection. J Immunol 168:4667–4673

Levadoux-Martin M, Gouble A, Jegou B, Vallet-Erdtmann V, Auriol J, Mercier P, Morello D (2003) Impaired gametogenesis in mice that overexpress the RNA-binding protein HuR. EMBO Rep 4:394–399

Lopez de Silanes I, Zhan M, Lal A, Yang X, Gorospe M (2004) Identification of a target RNA motif for RNA-binding protein HuR. Proc Natl Acad Sci USA 101:2987–2992

Lopez de Silanes I, Galban S, Martindale JL, Yang X, Mazan-Mamczarz K, Indig FE, Falco G, Zhan M, Gorospe M (2005) Identification and functional outcome of mRNAs associated with RNA-binding protein TIA-1. Mol Cell Biol 25:9520–9531

Lu JY, Sadri N, Schneider RJ (2006) Endotoxic shock in AUF1 knockout mice mediated by failure to degrade proinflammatory cytokine mRNAs. Genes Dev 20:3174–3184

Mijatovic T, Kruys V, Caput D, Defrance P, Huez G (1997) Interleukin-4 and -13 inhibit tumor necrosis factor-alpha mRNA translational activation in lipopolysaccharide-induced mouse macrophages. J Biol Chem 272:14394–14398

Mukherjee D, Gao M, O'Connor JP, Raijmakers R, Pruijn G, Lutz CS, Wilusz J (2002) The mammalian exosome mediates the efficient degradation of mRNAs that contain AU-rich elements. EMBO J 21:165–174

Neininger A, Kontoyiannis D, Kotlyarov A, Winzen R, Eckert R, Volk HD, Holtmann H, Kollias G, Gaestel M (2002) MK2 targets AU-rich elements and regulates biosynthesis of tumor necrosis factor and interleukin-6 independently at different post-transcriptional levels. J Biol Chem 277:3065–3068

Peifer C, Wagner G, Laufer S (2006) New approaches to the treatment of inflammatory disorders small molecule inhibitors of p38 MAP kinase. Curr Top Med Chem 6:113–149

Phillips K, Kedersha N, Shen L, Blackshear PJ, Anderson P (2004) Arthritis suppressor genes TIA-1 and TTP dampen the expression of tumor necrosis factor alpha, cyclooxygenase 2, and inflammatory arthritis. Proc Natl Acad Sci USA 101:2011–2016

Piecyk M, Wax S, Beck AR, Kedersha N, Gupta M, Maritim B, Chen S, Guey-
dan C, Kruys V, Streuli M, Anderson P (2000) TIA-1 is a translational
silencer that selectively regulates the expression of TNF-alpha. EMBO J
19:4154–4163

Rajasingh J, Bord E, Luedemann C, Asai J, Hamada H, Thorne T, Qin G,
Goukassian D, Zhu Y, Losordo DW, Kishore R (2006) IL-10-induced TNF-
alpha mRNA destabilization is mediated via IL-10 suppression of p38 MAP
kinase activation and inhibition of HuR expression. FASEB J 20:2112–
2114

Ramos SB, Stumpo DJ, Kennington EA, Phillips RS, Bock CB, Ribeiro-Neto
F, Blackshear PJ (2004) The CCCH tandem zinc-finger protein Zfp36l2 is
crucial for female fertility and early embryonic development. Development
131:4883–4893

Saklatvala J (2004) The p38 MAP kinase pathway as a therapeutic target in
inflammatory disease. Curr Opin Pharmacol 4:372–377

Shaw G, Kamen R (1986) A conserved AU sequence from the 3′ untranslated
region of GM-CSF mRNA mediates selective mRNA degradation. Cell
46:659–667

Stoecklin G, Anderson P (2006) Posttranscriptional mechanisms regulating the
inflammatory response. Adv Immunol 89:1–37

Stoecklin G, Mayo T, Anderson P (2006) ARE-mRNA degradation requires the
5′-3′ decay pathway. EMBO Rep 7:72–77

Stumpo DJ, Byrd NA, Phillips RS, Ghosh S, Maronpot RR, Castranio T, Meyers
EN, Mishina Y, Blackshear PJ (2004) Chorioallantoic fusion defects and
embryonic lethality resulting from disruption of Zfp36L1, a gene encoding
a CCCH tandem zinc finger protein of the Tristetraprolin family. Mol Cell
Biol 24:6445–6455

Sun L, Stoecklin G, Van Way S, Hinkovska-Galcheva V, Guo RF, Anderson
P, Shanley TP (2006) TTP/14-3-3 complex formation protects TTP from
dephosphorylation by protein phosphatase 2A and stabilizes TNF-alpha
mRNA. J Biol Chem 282:3766–3777

Tebo J, Der S, Frevel M, Khabar KS, Williams BR, Hamilton TA (2003) Heterogeneity in control of mRNA stability by AU-rich elements. J Biol Chem
278:12085–12093

Wilson GM, Brewer G (1999) The search for trans-acting factors controlling
messenger RNA decay. Prog Nucleic Acid Res Mol Biol 62:257–291

Wilson GM, Lu J, Sutphen K, Sun Y, Huynh Y, Brewer G (2003) Regulation of
A+U-rich element-directed mRNA turnover involving reversible phosphorylation of AUF1. J Biol Chem 278:33029–33038

Wilusz CJ, Gao M, Jones CL, Wilusz J, Peltz SW (2001) Poly(A)-binding proteins regulate both mRNA deadenylation and decapping in yeast cytoplasmic extracts. RNA 7:1416–1424

Xu N, Chen CY, Shyu AB (1997) Modulation of the fate of cytoplasmic mRNA by AU-rich elements: key sequence features controlling mRNA deadenylation and decay. Mol Cell Biol 17:4611–4621

Ernst Schering Foundation Symposium Proceedings, Vol. 4, pp. 59–68
DOI 10.1007/2789_2007_055
© Springer-Verlag Berlin Heidelberg
Published Online: 15 June 2007

Immunomodulatory Therapies: Challenges of Individualized Therapy Strategies

H.D. Volk[✉], B. Sawitzki, F. Kern, C. Höflich, R. Sabat, P. Reinke

Institute for Medical Immunology, Charité-University Medicine Berlin, Charitéplatz 1, 10117 Berlin, Germany
email: *hans-dieter.volk@charite.de*

Abstract. "Individualized therapy strategies" involve strategies that allow treatment to be guided by patient-specific conditions. For this, robust biomarkers are needed. Examples of biomarker-guided therapies already in use are the treatment of insulin-dependent diabetes (biomarker: blood glucose level) or the treatment of hypertension (biomarker: blood pressure). By contrast, most immunomodulatory therapies are given according to the patient's body weight or the patient's drug blood level rather than according to biomarkers indicating the patient's state of the immune system. Herein we report on new biomarker-guided studies in the immunosuppressive treatment of transplant patients and patients with autoimmune disease and we discuss its benefits and pitfalls.

1   Introduction

"Individualized therapy strategies" involve strategies that allow treatment to be guided by patient-specific conditions. To achieve these therapy strategies, two requirements need to be fulfilled: (1) subgroups with different response patterns have to be identified before the start of a particular treatment protocol to select the best therapy for the individual patient, (2) the therapeutic success/failure has to be monitored to adjust the therapy according to individual response as early as possible. To fulfill these criteria, robust biomarkers are needed.

Examples of individualized therapy strategies already in use are the medicinal treatment of diabetes or hypertension. In diabetic patients, the insulin dosage is adapted to the patient's blood glucose level. In the treatment of hypertension the dosage of the antihypertensive drug is adapted to the patient's blood pressure. By contrast, most immunomodulatory therapies are given according to the patient's body weight or the patient's drug blood level rather than according to biomarkers indicating the patient's state of the immune system.

To illustrate the first successful experiences with biomarker-guided studies, we will report on new biomarker-guided studies in the immunosuppressive treatment of transplant patients and patients with autoimmune disease and will discuss benefits and withdrawals. Concretely, three examples are presented and discussed:

1. Selecting transplant patients for an enhanced risk for cytomegalovirus (CMV) disease to improve antiviral management
2. Selecting the best immunosuppression for organ transplant patients
3. Monitoring the success of specific immunomodulatory therapies to select/adjust therapy in autoimmune patients

2   Selecting Transplant Patients on Enhanced Risk for CMV Disease to Improve Antiviral Management

CMV reactivation frequently occurs, but CMV disease only develops in cases of diminished T cell responses to control CMV reactivation (Quinnan et al. 1982). As immunosuppression in allotransplant patients so far does not discriminate between alloantigen specific and pathogen specific T cells, allotransplant patients are at high risk to develop life-threatening CMV disease (Fishman and Rubin 1998). Current standard treatment of CMV disease is antiviral therapy with ganciclovir. However, there is no correlation between initial viral load and response to ganciclovir, indicating that antiviral therapy alone may not be sufficient enough to control disease (Babel 2004).

Recently, Bunde et al. analyzed the T cells responses against the immunodominant CMV proteins pp65 and IE-1 in solid organ transplant patients and related them to the development of CMV disease (Bunde et al. 2005). This was done by usage of an epitope/HLA-independent flow cytometric method using protein spanning peptide pools of the pp65 and IE-1 protein (Kern et al. 1998). They could clearly demonstrate that, in contrast to pp65, the CMV IE-1 T cell response is associated with protection from CMV disease. The relevance of a strong IE-1-specific T cell response to control CMV disease development may be explained by the fact that following CMV reactivation—for instance by inflammation, stress, or some drugs—the IE-1 protein is the first protein expressed in monocyte precursor cells in the bone marrow (Stinski 1978; Döcke et al. 1994; Prösch et al. 1995). IE-1 protein-expressing precursor monocytes mature, become permissive to CMV replication, and migrate to the periphery, thus distributing the infectious virus (Waldman et al. 1995).

Consequences from these data are:

1. Antiviral strategies (e.g., long-term ganciclovir) should be accompanied by CMV-specific T cell monitoring.
2. Transplant patient with insufficient IE-1-specific T cell response are at enhanced risk for CMV disease, and their CMV load should be closely monitored to initiate preemptive antiviral therapy.

3. T cell-depleting strategies (e.g., Campath-1, ATG, but particularly anti-CD3) should be used very restrictive only if the CMV load is closely monitored.
4. Adoptive CMV targeting T cell therapy for severe CMV disease should include CMV IE-1-reactive cytotoxic T cells.

3   Selecting Best Immunosuppression for Organ Transplant Patients

Currently, standard immunosuppressive drugs suppress the immune system antigen independently. That is, alloantigen-specific as well as pathogen/tumor-specific responses are inhibited. Taken together with substrate specific actions, two types of side effects have to be taken care of when administering immunosuppressive drugs: inhibition of volitional immune responses and drug-specific side effects (for instance, renal dysfunction which may be caused by calcineurin inhibitors or rapamycin; post-transplant diabetes, which may be caused by FK506 or steroids). In order to minimize drug-specific side effects in allotransplant patients, standard treatment protocols usually contain combinations of various immunosuppressive drugs and, as mentioned earlier, the dosage is regulated by the patient's body weight or blood drug levels, respectively. However, except for the differentiation of high-risk patients, these protocols are used independently of patient-specific conditions. Therefore, among others, the following questions arise:

1. Does every patient need the same immunosuppression?
2. Which patients can be weaned from immunosuppression?

3.1   Does Every Patient Need the Same Immunosuppression?

The human T lymphocyte pool comprises everything from naïve T cells (including naïve alloreactive T cells), regulatory T cells, and memory T cells to environmental recall antigens and alloreactive memory T cells. By detecting alloreactive memory T cells using an interferon gamma (IFN-γ) ELISpot (enzyme-linked immunoabsorbent spot) assay, Nickel et al. recently showed that the occurrence of *pre*-transplant alloreactive memory T cells in "naïve" transplant recipients predicts negative short- and long-term graft function under conventional immunosuppression (Nickel et al. 2004). Furthermore, high frequencies of alloreactive T cells *after* transplantation showed a poorer 1-year creatinine clearance, indicating insufficient control of alloreactivity (Nickel et al. 2004). Importantly, memory T cell frequencies to multiple HLA-specificities (that is, panel reactive T cells, PRT) do not correlate with panel reactive antibody titers (Andree et al. 2006).

These data indicated that patients with high frequencies of alloreactive memory T cells prior to transplantation may benefit from specific elimination/functional inhibition of these T cells. Elimination of T cells can be achieved by (monoclonal) antibodies such as antithymocyte globulin (ATG) or Campath. However, incomplete depletion of almost all memory T cells results in lymphopenia-derived proliferation of alloreactive T cells and complete depletion results in severe inhibition of anti-infectious and antitumor competence (Ernst et al. 1999). Regarding functional inhibition of alloreactive T cells, except for calcineurin inhibitors, standard immunosuppressive drugs rather inhibit naïve than memory T cells. Calcineurin inhibitors are very potent inhibitors of both naïve and memory T cells. Therefore they cannot be spared for only those patients with high frequencies of alloreactive memory T cells. Furthermore, as with complete depletion, complete functional inhibition of the (memory) T cell pool would result in severe inhibition of anti-infectious and antitumor competence. In contrast to the elimination of T cell subsets regardless of their antigen specificity, the first clinical approaches to *selectively* eliminate *alloreactive* memory T cells have been conducted and the results are encouraging (N. Babel, L. Gabdrakhmanova, M. Hammer, C. Rosenberger, G. Bold, J.S. Juergensen, C. Schoenmann, H.D. Volk, and P. Reinke, manuscript in preparation).

3.2   Which Patients Can Be Weaned of Immunosuppression?

For many reasons, drug weaning in transplant patients is of importance. These reasons include (1) the reduction of short and long-term complications of immunosuppression, (2) the prevention of drug-induced graft injury, (3) a reduction of costs of long-term immunosuppressive therapy, and (4) the reduction of psychological reasons/compliance problems.

Drug weaning in transplant patients is possible because in most patients the rejection risk decreases with time due to tolerance mechanisms that are, however, only poorly understood. The first weaning trials show successful drug reduction in part of the patients but rejection episodes in others. In order to successfully wean transplant patients from immunosuppression, we need biomarkers guiding our protocols.

The EU integrated project "Reprogramming the immune system for the establishment of tolerance" (*www.risetfp6.org*) addresses these issues with goals to develop assays that will:

1. Identify drug weaning failure and/or tolerance induction before graft injury to introduce therapeutic adjustment on time (failure of tolerance)
2. Detect developing tolerance (success of tolerance) early

Ideally, biomarkers (that is rejection markers/tolerance markers) taken from noninvasive methods, e.g., using blood or urine, should fulfill these requirements.

With respect to rejection markers, Kotsch et al. could recently demonstrate that renal transplant patients with enhanced urinary cytotoxic T cell marker expression like granulysin are at enhanced risk of acute rejection, indicating the need for prolonged/intensified immunosuppression (Kotsch et al. 2004). With respect to tolerance markers, B. Sawitzki et al. studied the molecular signature of tolerance in renal transplant animal models and in humans using complementary DNA (cDNA) microarray and reverse transcriptase PCR (RT-PCR) techniques; by analyzing blood, a distinct marker set may be able to distinguish putative tolerant patients where minimizing of immunosuppression might be possible (B. Sawitzki, A. Bushell, U. Steger, N. Jones, K. Risch, A. Siepert, M. Lehmann, I. Schmitt-Knosalla, K. Vogt, I. Gebuhr, K. Wood, and H.D. Volk, manuscript in preparation).

4   Monitoring Success of Specific Immunomodulatory Therapies to Select/Adjust Therapy in Autoimmune Patients

Multiple sclerosis (MS) is an autoimmune disease in which T cells may play a central role (Wandinger et al. 2003). Interferon-β (IFN-β)

has become a worldwide standard in MS treatment, and its efficacy is well documented even if the mechanisms by which it changes the clinical course of MS are fairly unclear (Wandinger et al. 2003). As with virtually every drug, IFN-β is not free from side effects, and some patients do not respond to IFN-β. However, the clinical differentiation of therapeutic responder from nonresponder patients takes 6 to 12 months, revealing the need for a marker (set) to distinguish responder from nonresponder patients very early after onset of IFN-β thera5spy or, even better, before onset of treatment. By using cDNA microarray analysis of peripheral mononuclear cells from MS patients treated with IFN-β, Wandinger et al. could demonstrate the upregulation of tumor necrosis factor (TNF)-related apoptosis inducing ligand (TRAIL) messenger RNA (mRNA) in all patients (Wandinger et al. 2003). Importantly, as early as 4 weeks after onset of IFN-β therapy, so-called first-year responders had a significant higher TRAIL upregulation compared to first-year nonresponders. In the case of the formation of neutralizing anti-IFN-β autoantibodies, initial upregulation of TRAIL was abrogated (Wandinger et al. 2003). Additionally, baseline soluble TRAIL in sera of responder patients was significantly higher than in nonresponder patients, indicating that, even prior to therapy, responders might be distinguishable from nonresponders (Wandinger et al. 2003).

Psoriasis is another autoimmune disease where T cells may play a central pathogenetic role (Philipp et al. 2006). Alefacept is a fusion protein made of two human lymphocyte function antigen 3 proteins (LFA-3, CD58) and the Fc part of a human immunoglobulin G1. Alefacept binds to the CD2 molecule on T cells, inhibits T cell activation, and induces selective apoptosis and depletion of memory/effector T cells (Miller et al. 1993; Majeau et al. 1994; Meier et al. 1995). Consequently, Alefacept therapy has been successfully used in psoriatic patients (Lebwohl et al. 2003). However, measured by a Psoriasis Area and Severity Index (PASI) score reduction of more than 50%, responders significantly separated from nonresponders as late as 9 weeks after onset of therapy. By analyzing mRNA expression in peripheral blood mononuclear cells (PBMC) from treated patients, Gube et al. found a distinct marker set predicting response as early as 3 weeks after onset of therapy (K. Gube, M. Friedrich, I. Gebuhr, S. Philipp, R. Sabat, W. Sterry, H.D. Volk, and B. Sawitzki, manuscript submitted).

These data demonstrate that biomarkers can help to define subgroups with different response patterns prior to the start of or very early after the beginning of a particular treatment protocol. By this method, non-responder patients can be kept from therapies that would not be effective and could cause drug-specific side effects (such as depression with INF-β or lymphopenia with Alefacept).

5   Summary

The data presented at the Ernst Schering Foundation Scientific Symposium in October 2006 demonstrate that the identification of subgroups with distinct response pattern to immunomodulatory therapy is possible. Furthermore, the first biomarker-guided clinical trials show promise towards the development of more individualized therapy strategies. However, further validation strategies are necessary. Figure 1 summarizes the approach toward a more individualized immune therapy.

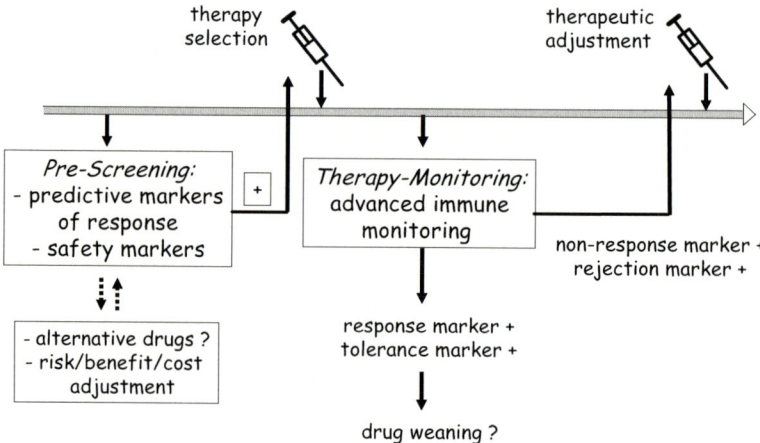

Fig. 1. Approach toward a more individualized immune therapy

References

Andree H, Nickel P, Nasiadko C, Hammer MH, Schonemann C, Pruss A, Volk HD, Reinke P (2006) Identification of dialysis patients with panel-reactive memory T cells before kidney transplantation using an allogeneic cell bank. J Am Soc Nephrol 17:573–580

Babel N, Gabdrakhmanova L, Juergensen JS, Eibl N, Hoerstrup J, Hammer M, Rosenberger C, Hoeflich C, Frei U, Rohde F, Volk HD, Reinke P (2004) Treatment of cytomegalovirus disease with valganciclovir in renal transplant recipients: a single center experience. Transplantation 27:283–285

Bunde T, Kirchner A, Hoffmeister B, Habedank D, Hetzer R, Cherepnev G, Proesch S, Reinke P, Volk HD, Lehmkuhl H, Kern F (2005) Protection from cytomegalovirus after transplantation is correlated with immediate early 1-specific CD8 T cells. J Exp Med 201:1031–1036

Döcke WD, Prosch S, Fietze E, Kimel V, Zuckermann H, Klug C, Syrbe U, Kruger DH, von Baehr R, Volk HD (1994) Cytomegalovirus reactivation and tumour necrosis factor. Lancet 343:268–269

Ernst B, Lee DS, Chang JM, Sprent J, Surh CD (1999) The peptide ligands mediating positive selection in the thymus control T cell survival and homeostatic proliferation in the periphery. Immunity 11:173–181

Fishman JA, Rubin RH (1998) Infection in organ-transplant recipients. N Engl J Med 338:1741–1751

Kern F, Surel IP, Brock C, Freistedt B, Radtke H, Scheffold A, Blasczyk R, Reinke P, Schneider-Mergener J, Radbruch A, Walden P, Volk HD (1998) T-cell epitope mapping by flow cytometry. Nat Med 4:975–978

Kotsch K, Mashreghi MF, Bold G, Tretow P, Beyer J, Matz M, Hoerstrup J, Pratschke J, Ding R, Suthanthiran M, Volk HD, Reinke P (2004) Enhanced granulysin mRNA expression in urinary sediment in early and delayed acute renal allograft rejection. Transplantation 77:1866–1875

Lebwohl M, Christophers E, Langley R, Ortonne JP, Roberts J, Griffiths CE (2003) Alefacept Clinical Study Group. An international, randomized, double-blind, placebo-controlled phase 3 trial of intramuscular alefacept in patients with chronic plaque psoriasis. Arch Dermatol 139:719–727

Majeau GR, Meier W, Jimmo B, Kioussis D, Hochman PS (1994) Mechanism of lymphocyte function-associated molecule 3-Ig fusion proteins inhibition of T cell responses: structure/function analysis in vitro and in human CD2 transgenic mice. J Immunol 152:2753–2767

Meier W, Gill A, Rogge M, Dabora R, Majeau GR, Oleson FB, Jones WE, Frazier D, Miatkowski K, Hochman PS (1995) Immunomodulation by LFA3TIP, an LFA-3/IgG1 fusion protein: cell line dependent glycosylation effects on pharmacokinetic and pharmacodynamic markers. Ther Immunol 2:159–171

Miller GT, Hochman PS, Meier W, Tizard R, Bixler SA, Rosa MD, Wallner BP (1993) Specific interaction of lymphocyte function-associated antigen 3 with CD2 can inhibit T cell responses. J Exp Med 178:211–222

Nickel P, Presber F, Bold G, Biti D, Schonemann C, Tullius SG, Volk HD, Reinke P (2004) Enzyme-linked immunosorbent spot assay for donor-reactive interferon-gamma-producing cells identifies T-cell presensitization and correlates with graft function at 6 and 12 months in renal-transplant recipients. Transplantation 78:1640–1646

Philipp S, Wolk K, Kreutzer S, Wallace E, Ludwig N, Roewert J, Hoflich C, Volk HD, Sterry W, Sabat R (2006) The evaluation of psoriasis therapy with biologics leads to a revision of the current view of the pathogenesis of this disorder. Expert Opin Ther Targets 10:817–831

Prösch S, Staak K, Stein J, Liebenthal C, Stamminger T, Volk HD, Kruger DH (1995) Stimulation of the human cytomegalovirus IE enhancer/promoter in HL-60 cells by TNFalpha is mediated via induction of NF-kappaB. Virology 208:197–206

Quinnan GV Jr, Kirmani N, Rook AH, Manischewitz JF, Jackson L, Moreschi G, Santos GW, Saral R, Burns WH (1982) Cytotoxic T cells in cytomegalovirus infection: HLA-restricted T-lymphocyte and non-T-lymphocyte cytotoxic responses correlate with recovery from cytomegalovirus infection in bone-marrow-transplant recipients. N Engl J Med 307:7–13

Stinski MF (1978) Sequence of protein synthesis in cells infected by human cytomegalovirus: early and late virus-induced polypeptides. J Virol 26:686–701

Waldman WJ, Knight DA, Huang EH, Sedmak DD (1995) Bidirectional transmission of infectious cytomegalovirus between monocytes and vascular endothelial cells: an in vitro model. J Infect Dis 171:263–272

Wandinger KP, Lunemann JD, Wengert O, Bellmann-Strobl J, Aktas O, Weber A, Grundstrom E, Ehrlich S, Wernecke KD, Volk HD, Zipp F (2003) TNF-related apoptosis inducing ligand (TRAIL) as a potential response marker for interferon-beta treatment in multiple sclerosis. Lancet 361:2036–2043

Ernst Schering Foundation Symposium Proceedings, Vol. 4, pp. 69–82
DOI 10.1007/2789_2007_039
© Springer-Verlag Berlin Heidelberg
Published Online: 15 June 2007

T Cell Therapies

S. Gottschalk(✉), C.M. Bollard, K.C. Straathof, C.U. Louis,
B. Savoldo, G. Dotti, M.K. Brenner, H.E. Heslop, C.M. Rooney

Center for Gene and Cell Therapy, Baylor College of Medicine, 6621 Fannin Street MC
3-3320, 77030 Houston, USA
email: *smg@bcm.edu*

Abstract. T cell therapies are increasingly used for the treatment of malignancies and viral-associated diseases. Initial studies focused on the use of unmanipulated T cell populations after allogeneic stem cell transplantation. More recently, the use of antigen-specific T cells has been explored. This chapter reviews the clinical experience with polyclonal Epstein-Barr virus (EBV)-specific cytotoxic T cells (CTL) for the treatment of EBV-associated malignancies. Strategies on how to improve the antitumor activity of EBV-specific CTL are being discussed. If effective, these strategies will have broad implications for T cell therapies for a range of human tumors with defined antigens.

1   Introduction

The use of donor lymphocyte infusions (DLI) for the successful treatment of hematological malignancies such as chronic myelogenous leukemia after hematopoietic stem cell transplantation (HSCT) has demonstrated the curative potential of T cell therapies (Kolb et al. 1990, 2004).
However, the use of DLI is limited by potentially fatal complications
such as graft-versus-host disease (GVHD) that arises from the presence
of alloreactive T cells. To overcome this limitation, strategies have been
developed to generate antigen-specific T cell products that are devoid
of alloreactivity.

Developing successful antigen-specific T cell therapies depends on
the availability of specific antigens as targets and efficient methods for
ex vivo T cell activation and expansion. Riddell et al. pioneered the use
of antigen-specific T cells to prevent cytomegalovirus (CMV) reactivation in HSCT recipients (Riddell et al. 1992). Donor-derived CD8-
positive T cell clones activated by coculture with CMV-infected, autologous fibroblasts and specific for the viral tegument proteins pp65 and
pp150 proved safe and protected HSCT recipients against the reactivation of CMV (Riddell et al. 1992; Peggs et al. 2003). Since then, studies have been performed with other antigen-specific T cells, including
Epstein-Barr virus (EBV)-specific T cells for the adoptive immunotherapy of EBV-associated diseases, melanoma antigen recognized by T
cells (MART-1)-specific or glycoprotein 100 (gp100)-specific T cells
for melanoma, and adenoviral-specific T cells (Rooney et al. 1998; Bollard et al. 2004a; Straathof et al. 2005a; Yee et al. 2002; Morgan et al.
2006). The results of these clinical trials indicate that antigen-specific
T cells are safe, and produce antiviral and antitumor effects. However,
T cells did not expand significantly in vivo unless the recipient's lymphoid compartment was depleted, as seen after HSCT, and only persisted if the infused T cell product contained CD4 T helper cells. Moreover, T cell escape mutants were observed when clonal or oligoclonal
T cell lines were infused (Yee et al. 2002; Gottschalk et al. 2001). These
results imply that therapeutic T cell products should target multiple antigens, and contain CD8-positive as well as CD4-positive T cells. In addition, robust *in vivo* T cell expansion most likely requires a lymphode-
pleted environment and/or the presence of antigen. In this chapter we

will highlight the successes and challenges of T cell therapies using EBV-associated malignancies as a model system.

2   EBV-Associated Malignancies

EBV is a latent γ-herpesvirus, and more than 90% of the world's population is EBV-positive. During primary infection, EBV establishes life-long latency in the memory B cell compartment, and the number of latently infected B cells within an individual remains stable over years (Cohen 2000). Healthy individuals mount a vigorous humoral and cellular immune response to primary infection (Rickinson and Kieff 2001). Although EBV-specific antibodies neutralize virus infectivity, the cellular immune response, consisting of CD4-positive and CD8-positive T cells, is essential for controlling primary and latent EBV infection.

All EBV-associated malignancies are associated with the virus' latent cycle (Hsu and Glaser 2000). In type I latency, which is found in EBV-positive Burkitt's lymphoma, only Epstein-Barr nuclear antigen 1 (EBNA1), EBV-encoded small nuclear RNAs (EBERs), and the BamHI-A rightward transcripts (BARTs) are expressed. Type II latency, characterized by EBNA1, latent membrane proteins (LMP1, LMP2), EBERs, and BARTs expression, is found in EBV-positive Hodgkin's disease, nasopharyngeal carcinoma (NPC), and peripheral T/natural killer (NK) cell lymphomas. While malignancies associated with type I and II latency occur in individuals with minimal or no immune dysfunction, type III latency is associated with malignancies in severely immunocompromised patients. It is characterized by the expression of the entire array of EBV latency genes, being EBNAs 1, 2, 3A, 3B, 3C, leader protein (LP), LMP1, LMP2, EBERs, and BARTs. This pattern of gene expression is found in EBV-associated lymphoproliferative disease (EBV-LPD) after HSCT or solid organ transplant (SOT), and in EBV-associated lymphomas occurring in patients with congenital immunodeficiency or human immunodeficiency virus (HIV) infection. In addition, type III latency is found in lymphoblastoid cell lines (LCL), which can be readily prepared by infecting B cells in vitro with EBV and are instrumental in the generation of EBV-specific cytotoxic T lymphocytes (CTL) for the prophylaxis and therapy of EBV-LPD.

3   Adoptive Immunotherapy
for EBV Latency Type II Malignancies

3.1   Adoptive Immunotherapy for EBV-LPD After HSCT

Unmanipulated donor T cells have been used to treat HSCT recipients with established EBV-LPD with variable success, likely reflecting differences in EBV-specific T cell precursor frequencies in the infused T cell lines and/or a better outcome with early diagnosis and treatment (Papadopoulos et al. 1994; Lucas et al. 1998; Porter et al. 1994; Heslop et al. 1994; O'Reilly et al. 1997). Moreover, the use of donor T cells is limited by GVHD, a potential life-threatening complication. Two strategies have been developed to reduce the risk of GVHD. One strategy discussed in Sect. 5 relies on the transduction of T cells with a 'suicide gene' so that cell death can be induced if GVHD develops. The second strategy to prevent GVHD after donor T cell infusion is to infuse EBV-specific T cell lines, which lack alloreactivity. EBV-specific T cells can readily be generated from EBV-seropositive donors and the generated T cell lines are polyclonal and contain not only CD8-positive but also CD4-positive EBV-specific T cells (Rooney et al. 1998; Heslop et al. 1996). We have administered donor-derived EBV-specific CTL as prophylaxis or therapy for EBV-LPD in high-risk HSCT recipients. Infused CTL (1) were safe and induced no significant GVHD, (2) expanded by several orders of magnitude *in vivo*, (3) survived for up to 7 years after infusion, and (4) reduced the high virus load that was present in about 20% of patients at the time of infusion (Rooney et al. 1998; Heslop et al. 1996). EBV-specific CTL also appeared to prevent development of EBV-LPD, since none of 60 patients who received prophylactic CTL developed this malignancy, compared with 11.5% of controls. Six of seven patients who received CTL as treatment for EBV-LPD achieved complete remissions (Rooney et al. 1998; Pakakasama et al. 2004). The patient who did not respond illustrates one of the problems of immunotherapy: mutation of CTL target epitopes on tumor cells allowing escape from T cell recognition. The therapy failure was caused by a deletion in the EBV-derived EBNA3B gene in the tumor that removed immunodominant epitopes, thereby causing tumor-cell resistance to CTL killing (Gottschalk et al. 2001).

3.2 Adoptive Immunotherapy for EBV-LPD After SOT

The success of donor-derived EBV-specific CTL as prophylaxis and treatment of EBV-LPD after HSCT has resulted in the development of adoptive immunotherapy strategies for EBV-LPD after SOT. Since the majority of EBV-LPD after SOT are of recipient origin and donors are not HLA matched, the use of donor-derived EBV-specific T cells is of limited value. Therefore the use of autologous or partially HLA-matched EBV-specific CTL has been explored (Savoldo et al. 2006; Haque et al. 2002, 1998; Khanna et al. 1999). These studies demonstrated that infused EBV-specific CTL (1) did not cause graft rejection, (2) increased EBV-specific cellular immune responses *in vivo*, and (3) had antiviral and antitumor effects. However, in contrast to HSCT recipients, the infused EBV-specific CTL persisted only transiently and did not expand significantly, which may indicate that CTL do not persist because of ongoing immunosuppression and that CTL expansion is limited in patients who have a lymphocyte compartment close to or at steady state.

4 Adoptive Immunotherapy for EBV Latency Type III Malignancies

Hodgkin's disease and NPC are associated with EBV latency type II. In contrast to EBV-LPD, only a limited number of EBV-derived antigens, EBNA1, LMP1, and LMP2, are present in EBV-positive Hodgkin's disease and NPC. Nevertheless, the viral antigens provide targets for the adoptive immunotherapy with EBV-specific CTL.

4.1 Hodgkin's Disease

Autologous EBV-specific CTL have been given to patients with EBV-positive Hodgkin's disease with multiple relapses or with minimal residual disease after autologous HSCT (Bollard et al. 2004a; Roskrow et al. 1998). No immediate toxicities were seen. Infused CTL localized to a malignant pleural effusion in one patient and were detected at the tumor site of another patient at autopsy. Immunological studies showed an increase of LMP2-specific and EBV-specific cellular immunity after

CTL infusion, and gene-marked CTL were detected for up to 12 months. Eight patients with advanced disease remained alive for 2–20 months after CTL infusion. One patient with stable disease received an allogeneic HSCT and is in remission 4½ years after CTL infusion. Two patients are in complete remission 9–27 months after CTL infusion. These results indicate that infused EBV-specific CTL in Hodgkin's disease patients (1) are well tolerated, (2) persist for up to 12 months after infusion, (3) enhance EBV-specific immunity, and (4) localize to tumor sites.

4.2 Nasopharyngeal Carcinoma

Three groups of investigators have reported on the use of autologous EBV-specific CTL for the adoptive immunotherapy of patients with recurrent/refractory NPC (Straathof et al. 2005a; Chua et al. 2001; Comoli et al. 2005). In one study, four NPC patients with advanced disease were infused and an increase in EBV-specific CTL precursor frequency was observed, as well as a reduction in plasma EBV-DNA levels. No decrease in tumor size was observed; however, all patients had a large tumor burden (Chua et al. 2001). In the second study, ten patients were treated with EBV-specific CTL and in six of the ten patients control of disease progression was achieved (Comoli et al. 2005). Our group has evaluated the use of EBV-specific CTL in 13 patients; 7 of them had recurrent/refractory disease, while 6 had advanced-stage disease at presentation but were in remission at the time of CTL infusion. Of the 7 patients with recurrent disease, 2 patients are in biopsy-proven complete remission (CR) after CTL, 1 had a partial response for 12 months, 2 had stable disease, and 2 had no response (Straathof et al. 2005a).

The clinical experience with EBV-specific CTL for Hodgkin's disease and NPC indicates that EBV is a legitimate target for T cell targeted therapies. However, EBV-specific CTL were less effective for the treatment of Hodgkin's disease and NPC than for the treatment of EBV-LPD. One explanation for this failure is that EBV-specific CTL generated with LCL are dominated by clones reactive to EBV proteins not expressed in Hodgkin's disease or NPC. Furthermore, EBV-specific CTL did not expand significantly after infusion, indicating that CTL expansion may be limited in patients in which the lymphocyte compartment is close to steady state. In addition, EBV-specific CTL might be inhibited at the tumor site by immune-evasion strategies employed by the malignant cells of Hodgkin's disease and NPC. Thus, improvement of EBV-specific CTL therapy for Hodgkin's disease and NPC will require strategies to (1) expand CTL specific for EBV proteins expressed in these malignancies, (2) create a favorable environment for T cell expansion in vivo, and (3) genetically modify CTL to render them resistant to the inhibitory tumor environment.

5 Improving T Cell Therapies for EBV-Associated Malignancies

5.1 LMP-1-Specific and LMP2-Specific T Cells

In Hodgkin's disease and NPC, three EBV proteins are expressed: EBNA1, LMP1, and LMP2. Of these, only LMP1 and LMP2 are good targets for adoptive immunotherapy approaches, since EBNA1 is mainly presented on MHC class II molecules. Several groups have developed strategies to generate LMP1-specific and LMP2-specific CTL with autologous dendritic cells (DC) as antigen-presenting cells (APC) expressing LMP2, functionally inactive LMP1 or an "LMP1-LMP2 polyepitope" (Gahn et al. 2001; Gottschalk et al. 2003; Duraiswamy et al. 2004). We have developed a "polyclonal CTL expansion protocol" in which LMP2-specific CTL are initially activated with DC expressing LMP2, and subsequently expanded with LMP2 overexpressing LCL (Bollard et al. 2004b). The safety and efficacy of LMP2-specific CTL for EBV-positive Hodgkin's and non-Hodgkin's lymphoma are currently being evaluated in a phase I clinical trial (Bollard et al. 2005). So far 14 patients have been infused, and we have observed an increase in the frequency of infused CTL in 8 out of 10 evaluable patients. In addition, LMP2-specific CTL were detected at tumor sites. Out of 8 patients with detectable disease at the time of CTL infusion, 5 had clinical responses. These results indicate that LMP2-specific CTL are safe, accumulate at tumor sites, and have antitumor activity.

5.2 Lymphodepletion

EBV-specific CTL expanded *in vivo* by orders of magnitude only in HSCT recipients, indicating that the CTL expansion rate may be limited in patients in which the lymphocyte compartment is close to steady state. Dudley et al. reported the use of fludarabine and cyclophosphamide to create a proliferative environment prior T cell transfer (Dudley et al. 2002; Dudley and Rosenberg 2003). Selective expansion of infused T cells might also be obtained by using monoclonal antibodies (MAbs) to deplete the lymphoid compartment. We are currently evaluating MAbs directed to the common leukocyte antigen CD45. In murine studies administration of CD45 MAbs depleted all leukocyte lineages (Wulf et al. 2003). This depletion was prolonged only in lymphoid lineages, as neutrophils began to recover 48 h after injection. By contrast, marrow progenitor cells, which express CD45 at low levels, were spared. For our clinical studies, we have chosen a pair of rat IgG1 antibodies that can fix human complement and induce antibody-dependent cellular cytotoxicity, while having a short half-life that permits rapid subsequent infusion of the CTL. CD45 MAbs were initially evaluated in the clinic as part of an ablative preparative regimen for a stem cell allograft. The MAbs were well tolerated at a dose of 400 μg/kg per day for 4 days, producing more than 95% depletion of peripheral blood lymphocytes, predominantly T cells and NK cells (Krance et al. 2003). They reduced neutrophil counts by more than 90%, but, as anticipated, marrow sampling showed retention of CD34$^+$ progenitor cells, followed by partial neutrophil recovery within 48 h of the last dose of antibody. We are currently evaluating the use of CD45 MAbs in phase I clinical trials to transiently lymphodeplete patients with EBV-positive malignancies prior to infusion of EBV-specific or LMP2-specific CTL. In several patients we have observed enhanced T cell expansion after infusion in comparison to CTL infusions in the same patients without lymphodepletion (Louis et al. 2006).

5.3 Genetic Modification

5.3.1 Rendering CTL Resistant to the Immunosuppressive Tumor Environment

In vivo EBV-specific T cells often encounter an immunosuppressive environment created by tumor cells. This includes the presence of inhibitory cytokines secreted by tumor cells, such as transforming growth factor β (TGF-β) and/or apoptosis-inducing molecules such as Fas ligand (FasL), which are present on the cell surface of tumor cells. In preclinical studies, EBV-specific CTL have been genetically modified to render them resistant to TGF-β by expression of a dominant negative TGF-β type II receptor (Bollard et al. 2002). In addition, EBV-specific CTL expressing a small interfering RNA (siRNA) against Fas were shown to be resistant to FasL-induced apoptosis (Dotti et al. 2005). While these "proof of principle" studies were performed *ex vivo*, current efforts are focused on showing in preclinical animal models and/or phase I clinical trials that these genetic modifications translate into greater antitumor activity of adoptively transferred EBV-specific CTL *in vivo*.

5.3.2   Genetic Safety Switches

Genetic safety switches to selectively kill infused T cells to prevent serious side effects will make current T cell therapies, such as DLI, safer. In addition, safety switches will also reduce the risk:benefit ratio of evaluating genetically modified T cells in clinical trials. Several genetic safety switches have been developed, and the most widely used "switch" takes advantage of the herpes simplex virus derived thymidine kinase (HSV-tk), which phosphorylates acyclovir, valacyclovir or ganciclovir to toxic nucleosides. In a phase I clinical trial, donor-derived T cells transduced with the HSV-*tk* gene were infused into HSCT recipients (Bonini et al. 1997). Six patients developed GVHD and four had a complete resolution of GVHD after ganciclovir treatment. One drawback of this approach is the inherent immunogenicity of HSV-*tk* (Berger et al. 2006). Therefore, genetic safety switches using nonimmunogenic human components such as CD20, inducible Fas, or caspase, have been developed and successfully tested in preclinical animal models (Straathof et al. 2005b; Serafini et al. 2004; Thomis et al. 2001).

5.3.3   Expanding the Use of EBV-Specific CTL
          to EBV-Negative Malignancies

EBV-specific CTL are an attractive "T cell therapy platform" to target other malignancies since they (1) can be generated reliably from EBV-seropositive donors for clinical use, and (2) have an excellent safety record in clinical studies. One strategy to target EBV-specific CTL to non-EBV antigens is to express chimeric antigen receptors (CARs) on EBV-specific CTL (Pule et al. 2003; Eshhar et al. 1993). CARs are fusions between an antigen-recognizing ectodomain and a signaling endodomain, most commonly connecting the antigen-recognition properties of a monoclonal antibody with the endodomain of the CD3-ζ chain of the T cell receptor. CARs recognize tumor cells in an MHC-unrestricted manner and are therefore immune to some of the major mechanisms by which tumors avoid MHC-restricted T cell recognition, such as downregulation of HLA class I molecules and defects in antigen processing. We have shown in preclinical studies that EBV-specific CTL expressing CARs specific for antigens such as GD2a, CD30, and HER2, kill autologous EBV-positive target cells as well tumor cells expressing the CAR-specific antigen (Rossig et al. 2002). A clinical trial using EBV-specific CTL expressing GD2a-specific CARs is currently being conducted.

6   Conclusions

T cell therapies are increasingly used for the treatment of malignancies and viral-associated diseases. The adoptive immunotherapy with EBV-specific CTL is an effective strategy after HSCT to reconstitute EBV-specific immunity and prevent or treat EBV-LPD. For other EBV-associated malignancies, the use of EBV-specific CTL is so far less effective; however, the results are sufficiently encouraging to justify continued exploration of this approach. New strategies are being developed to enhance the antitumor activity of EBV-specific CTL by targeting CTL to subdominant EBV antigens, and by genetically modifying CTL to render them resistant to the immunosuppressive tumor environment. If effective, these strategies will have broad implications for T cell therapies for a range of human tumors with defined antigens.

Acknowledgements. The authors were supported by NIH grants PO1 CA94237 and the GCRC at Baylor College of Medicine (grant RR00188). S.G. is the recipient of a Doris Duke Clinical Scientist Development Award. H.E.H is the recipient of a Doris Duke Distinguished Clinical Scientist Award.

References

Berger C, Flowers ME, Warren EH, Riddell SR (2006) Analysis of transgene-specific immune responses that limit the in vivo persistence of adoptively transferred HSV-TK-modified donor T cells after allogeneic hematopoietic cell transplantation. Blood 107:2294–2302

Bollard CM, Rossig C, Calonge MJ et al. (2002) Adapting a transforming growth factor beta-related tumor protection strategy to enhance antitumor immunity. Blood 99:3179–3187

Bollard CM, Aguilar L, Straathof KC et al. (2004a) Cytotoxic T lymphocyte therapy for Epstein-Barr virus+ Hodgkin's disease. J Exp Med 200:1623–1633

Bollard CM, Straathof K, Huls MH et al. (2004b) The generation and characterization of LMP2-specific CTLs for use as adoptive transfer from patients with relapsed EBV-positive Hodgkin disease. J Immunother 27:317–327

Bollard CM, Buza E, Huls HM et al. (2005) The use of autologous LMP2-specific CTL for the treatment of relapsed EBV-positive Hodgkin disease and non-Hodgkin lymphoma. Blood (ASH Annual Meeting Abstr) 106:773

Bonini C, Ferrari G, Verzeletti S et al. (1997) HSV-TK gene transfer into donor lymphocytes for control of allogeneic graft-versus-leukemia. Science 276:1719–1724

Chua D, Huang J, Zheng B et al. (2001) Adoptive transfer of autologous Epstein-Barr virus-specific cytotoxic T cells for nasopharyngeal carcinoma. Int J Cancer 94:73–80

Cohen JI (2000) Epstein-Barr virus infection. N Engl J Med 343:481–492

Comoli P, Pedrazzoli P, Maccario R et al. (2005) Cell therapy of stage IV nasopharyngeal carcinoma with autologous Epstein-Barr virus-targeted cytotoxic T lymphocytes. J Clin Oncol 23:8942–8949

Dotti G, Savoldo B, Pule M et al. (2005) Human cytotoxic T lymphocytes with reduced sensitivity to Fas-induced apoptosis. Blood 105:4677–4684

Dudley ME, Rosenberg SA (2003) Adoptive-cell-transfer therapy for the treatment of patients with cancer. Nat Rev Cancer 3:666–675

Dudley ME, Wunderlich JR, Robbins PF et al. (2002) Cancer regression and autoimmunity in patients after clonal repopulation with antitumor lymphocytes. Science 298:850–854

Duraiswamy J, Bharadwaj M, Tellam J et al. (2004) Induction of therapeutic T-cell responses to subdominant tumor-associated viral oncogene after immunization with replication-incompetent polyepitope adenovirus vaccine. Cancer Res 64:1483–1489

Eshhar Z, Waks T, Gross G, Schindler DG (1993) Specific activation and targeting of cytotoxic lymphocytes through chimeric single chains consisting of antibody-binding domains and the gamma or zeta subunits of the immunoglobulin and T-cell receptors. Proc Natl Acad Sci USA 90:720–724

Gahn B, Siller-Lopez F, Pirooz AD et al. (2001) Adenoviral gene transfer into dendritic cells efficiently amplifies the immune response to LMP2A antigen: a potential treatment strategy for Epstein-Barr virus-positive Hodgkin's lymphoma. Int J Cancer 93:706–713

Gottschalk S, Ng CY, Perez M et al. (2001) An Epstein-Barr virus deletion mutant associated with fatal lymphoproliferative disease unresponsive to therapy with virus-specific CTLs. Blood 97:835–843

Gottschalk S, Edwards OL, Sili U et al. (2003) Generating CTLs against the subdominant Epstein-Barr virus LMP1 antigen for the adoptive immunotherapy of EBV-associated malignancies. Blood 101:1905–1912

Haque T, Amlot PL, Helling N et al. (1998) Reconstitution of EBV-specific T cell immunity in solid organ transplant recipients. J Immunol 160:6204–6209

Haque T, Wilkie GM, Taylor C et al. (2002) Treatment of Epstein-Barr-virus-positive post-transplantation lymphoproliferative disease with partly HLA-matched allogeneic cytotoxic T cells. Lancet 360:436–442

Heslop HE, Brenner MK, Rooney CM (1994) Donor T cells to treat EBV-associated lymphoma. N Engl J Med 331:679–680

Heslop HE, Ng CY, Li C et al. (1996) Long-term restoration of immunity against Epstein-Barr virus infection by adoptive transfer of gene-modified virus-specific T lymphocytes. Nat Med 2:551–555

Hsu JL, Glaser SL (2000) Epstein-Barr virus-associated malignancies: epidemiologic patterns and etiologic implications. Crit Rev Oncol Hematol 34:27–53

Khanna R, Bell S, Sherritt M et al. (1999) Activation and adoptive transfer of Epstein-Barr virus-specific cytotoxic T cells in solid organ transplant patients with posttransplant lymphoproliferative disease. Proc Natl Acad Sci USA 96:10391–10396

Kolb HJ, Mittermuller J, Clemm C et al. (1990) Donor leukocyte transfusions for treatment of recurrent chronic myelogenous leukemia in marrow transplant patients. Blood 76:2462–2465

Kolb HJ, Simoes B, Schmid C (2004) Cellular immunotherapy after allogeneic stem cell transplantation in hematologic malignancies. Curr Opin Oncol 16:167–173

Krance RA, Kuehnle I, Rill DR et al. (2003) Hematopoietic and immunomodulatory effects of lytic CD45 monoclonal antibodies in patients with hematologic malignancy. Biol Blood Marrow Transplant 9:273–281

Louis CU, Straathof K, Torrano V et al. (2006) Treatment of Epstein-Barr virus-positive nasopharyngeal carcinoma with adoptively transferred cytotoxic T cells. 97th AACR Annual Meeting Abstr 4000

Lucas KG, Burton RL, Zimmerman SE et al. (1998) Semiquantitative Epstein-Barr virus (EBV) polymerase chain reaction for the determination of patients at risk for EBV-induced lymphoproliferative disease after stem cell transplantation. Blood 91:3654–3661

Morgan RA, Dudley ME, Wunderlich JR et al. (2006) Cancer regression in patients after transfer of genetically engineered lymphocytes. Science 314:126–129

O'Reilly RJ, Small TN, Papadopoulos E et al. (1997) Biology and adoptive cell therapy of Epstein-Barr virus-associated lymphoproliferative disorders in recipients of marrow allografts. Immunol Rev 157:195–216

Pakakasama S, Eames GM, Morriss MC et al. (2004) Treatment of Epstein-Barr virus lymphoproliferative disease after hematopoietic stem-cell transplantation with hydroxyurea and cytotoxic T-cell lymphocytes. Transplantation 78:755–757

Papadopoulos EB, Ladanyi M, Emanuel D et al. (1994) Infusions of donor leukocytes to treat Epstein-Barr virus-associated lymphoproliferative disorders after allogeneic bone marrow transplantation. N Engl J Med 330:1185–1191

Peggs KS, Verfuerth S, Pizzey A et al. (2003) Adoptive cellular therapy for early cytomegalovirus infection after allogeneic stem-cell transplantation with virus-specific T-cell lines. Lancet 362:1375–1377

Porter DL, Orloff GJ, Antin JH (1994) Donor mononuclear cell infusions as therapy for B-cell lymphoproliferative disorder following allogeneic bone marrow transplant. Transplant Sci 4:12–14

Pule M, Finney H, Lawson A (2003) Artificial T-cell receptors. Cytotherapy 5:211–226

Rickinson AB, Kieff E (2001) Epstein-Barr virus. In: Knipe DM, Howley PM (eds) Fields virology. Lippincott Williams and Williams, Philadelphia, pp 2575–2628

Riddell SR, Watanabe KS, Goodrich JM et al. (1992) Restoration of viral immunity in immunodeficient humans by the adoptive transfer of T cell clones. Science 257:238–241

Rooney CM, Smith CA, Ng CY et al. (1998) Infusion of cytotoxic T cells for the prevention and treatment of Epstein-Barr virus-induced lymphoma in allogeneic transplant recipients. Blood 92:1549–1555

Roskrow MA, Suzuki N, Gan Y et al. (1998) Epstein-Barr virus (EBV)-specific cytotoxic T lymphocytes for the treatment of patients with EBV-positive relapsed Hodgkin's disease. Blood 91:2925–2934

Rossig C, Bollard CM, Nuchtern JG, Rooney CM, Brenner MK (2002) Epstein-Barr virus-specific human T lymphocytes expressing antitumor chimeric T-cell receptors: potential for improved immunotherapy. Blood 99:2009–2016

Savoldo B, Goss JA, Hammer MM et al. (2006) Treatment of solid organ transplant recipients with autologous Epstein Barr virus-specific cytotoxic T lymphocytes (CTLs). Blood 108:2942–2949

Serafini M, Manganini M, Borleri G et al. (2004) Characterization of CD20-transduced T lymphocytes as an alternative suicide gene therapy approach for the treatment of graft-versus-host disease. Hum Gene Ther 15:63–76

Straathof KC, Bollard CM, Popat U et al. (2005a) Treatment of nasopharyngeal carcinoma with Epstein-Barr virus—specific T lymphocytes. Blood 105:1898–1904

Straathof KC, Pule MA, Yotnda P et al. (2005b) An inducible caspase 9 safety switch for T-cell therapy. Blood 105:4247–4254

Thomis DC, Marktel S, Bonini C et al. (2001) A Fas-based suicide switch in human T cells for the treatment of graft-versus-host disease. Blood 97:1249–1257

Wulf GG, Luo KL, Goodell MA, Brenner MK (2003) Anti-CD45-mediated cytoreduction to facilitate allogeneic stem cell transplantation. Blood 101:2434–2439

Yee C, Thompson JA, Byrd D et al. (2002) Adoptive T cell therapy using antigen-specific CD8+ T cell clones for the treatment of patients with metastatic melanoma: in vivo persistence, migration, and antitumor effect of transferred T cells. Proc Natl Acad Sci USA 99:16168–16173

Ernst Schering Foundation Symposium Proceedings, Vol. 4, pp. 83–106
DOI 10.1007/2789_2007_040
© Springer-Verlag Berlin Heidelberg
Published Online: 15 June 2007

The Future of Antibody Therapy

R. Buelow$^{(\boxtimes)}$, W. van Schooten

Therapeutic Human Polyclonals Inc., 2105 Landings Drive, 94043, Mountain View, USA
email: *rolandbuelow@aol.com*

Abstract. Antibodies have been used successfully as therapeutics for over 100 years. The successful development of therapeutic human(ized) monoclonal antibodies (mAbs) in the last 20 years has demonstrated the potency of mAbs but also revealed some of their limitations. Studies in animals and humans demonstrated that it is possible to overcome some of these limitations using mixtures of mAbs or polyclonal antibody (pAb) preparations. pAbs from human and animal plasma are efficacious and safe therapeutics for the treatment of many diseases. Novel technologies are being developed for the production of human pAbs in genetically engineered animals. Immunization of such animals should allow the production of effective and safe high-titer antibody preparations for the treatment of infectious diseases, cancer, and autoimmunity.

1   Historical Perspective

Antibodies have been used successfully as drugs since the 1890s, when it was found that polyclonal antiserum taken from animals could treat life-threatening infections in humans (Casadevall and Scharff 1994, 1995; Buchwald and Pirofski 2003). By the 1920s, "serum therapy" had gained widespread use in treating many infectious diseases including pneumonia, meningitis, scarlet fever, whooping cough, anthrax, botulism, tetanus, diphtheria, measles, mumps, and chickenpox. However, this use was ultimately limited by a side effect called serum sickness, an unwanted immune response mounted against the nonhuman proteins within the antiserum. The introduction of the antibiotics sulfonamide, in 1935, and penicillin, in 1942, further diminished use of serum therapy for treating many infectious diseases. Even with these limitations, animal-derived polyclonal therapy continued to be used to treat numerous diseases, and is still used today as standard care for treating botulinum toxin exposure, venomous bites, certain drug overdoses, and immune suppression in organ graft recipients.

A significant advance in antibody research occurred in 1975 when Kohler and Milstein described a technology to prepare and produce monoclonal antibodies (mAbs) in vitro (Kohler and Milstein 1975). For the first time, researchers and clinicians were able to replicate and harness the therapeutic powers of single antibodies created by the immune system.

Although mAbs promised to be biotechnology's "magic bullet," by the early 1990s all but one of 49 tested in clinical trials had failed. The first generation of mouse-derived monoclonals suffered serious side effects due to an unwanted immune reaction in humans referred to as a "human anti-mouse antibody response" (HAMA) (Badger et al. 1987; Khazaeli et al. 1994; Lee et al. 1998). This response, characterized by fever, chills, arthralgia and life-threatening anaphylaxis was identical to the serum sickness observed some 50 years earlier with animal antisera. To realize the full promise of monoclonals, scientists needed a technology to "humanize" animal-derived antibodies and make them less immunogenic and safer.

Advances in genetic engineering in the late 1980s provided the technology to humanize mouse-derived mAbs including chimerization, complementarity-determining region (CDR) grafting, display libraries, and human immunoglobulin transgenic mice (Adams and Weiner 2005; Wu and Senter 2005; Hoogenboom 2005; Lonberg 2005; Holliger and Hudson 2005). These approaches have created substantially human mAbs that have proven themselves effective in human patients with minimal side effects and long half-lives. The humanization of monoclonals has been the springboard for launching antibodies as a clinically acceptable class of therapeutics. Even though major pharmaceutical firms were initially reluctant to adopt mAb therapy, most have now one or more mAbs in clinical studies, clearly demonstrating that antibody therapy has come of age. Currently, approximately 150 humanized mAbs are being tested in clinical trials, and 18 antibody drugs were approved by the FDA in the last 10 years, generating revenue in excess of US $10 billion in 2005.

The potential future of mAbs and their derivatives (single chain antibodies, antibody fragments, conjugates with toxins/radionucleotides/enzymes) has been reviewed in a number of recent publications (Adams and Weiner 2005; Wu and Senter 2005; Hoogenboom 2005; Lonberg 2005; Holliger and Hudson 2005). Here we will contemplate the limitations of currently used monoclonal and polyclonal antibody therapies and discuss novel developments of therapeutic oligoclonal (mixtures of monoclonals) and polyclonal antibody preparations.

2 Limitations of Current Monoclonal and Polyclonal Antibody Therapy

Today, 18 mAb therapies have been approved for human use and a large number of mAbs are in clinical development for cancer and inflammatory diseases. For these indications, development of therapeutic mAbs has a high success rate, and roughly 20% of mAbs entering clinical trial obtained approval from the FDA (Reichert et al. 2005; Reichert and Dewitz 2006). In contrast, mAbs as anti-infective agents have been shown to be more difficult to develop. Out of 46 anti-infective mAbs tested in the clinic, only one, palivizumab, was approved as a prophylaxis of respiratory syncytial virus infection in high-risk pediatric patients (Reichert and Dewitz 2006).

Antibodies mediate protection by a variety of mechanisms, including blockade of receptor–ligand interactions, agglutination and immobilization, viral and toxin neutralization, antibody-mediated cellular cytotoxicity (ADCC), complement-dependent cytotoxicity (CDC), and opsonization. Because mAbs are limited to binding a single epitope on a single antigen, they are ideal for some functions but less optimal for others. MAbs are best suited for blocking ligand docking to a receptor. For example, treatment of rheumatoid arthritis by blocking a critical inflammatory cytokine, tumor necrosis factor (TNF)-α, with infliximab ameliorates disease by suppression of the inflammatory response (Finckh et al. 2006). Likewise, antagonizing CD25, the interleukin (IL)-2 receptor, with basiliximab or daclizumab has also proven effective in treating allograft rejection (Church 2003). In such cases, the monoclonal drug is effective because it blocks the cytokine from docking and stimulating its receptor. The narrow specificity of monoclonals is also exploited by the clot-busting drug abciximab, which is active only against the pro-thrombic factor IIb/IIIb (Ringleb 2006).

Although human mAb drugs have been used to treat cancer, the effectiveness of such therapies is limited by the capacity of single mAbs to trigger immune effector functions that lead to target cell death. Many anti-tumor mAbs have been shown to mediate ADCC in vitro, but the relevance of this mechanism of action to clinical efficacy has not been proven. On the other hand, several groups have recently shown that the efficacy of rituximab is substantially greater in patients with high responder' Fc-receptor polymorphism (Cartron et al. 2002; Weng and Levy 2003). These findings indicate that interaction between the antibody Fc domain and the Fc-receptor underlie at least some of the clinical benefit of rituximab, and imply the importance of ADCC.

Similarly, the ability of anti-tumor mAbs to elicit CDC is limited by the low density of some target molecules on the surface of cancer cells. Since cancer is a disease characterized by a heterogeneous population of cells, it is rare to find a single target that is expressed in high abundance on all cancer cells. Monoclonal therapies such as rituximab, which targets CD20, and trastuzumab, which targets HER2, are effective in targeting some cells, but tumors expressing lower levels of the target protein escape from the monoclonal therapy (Golay et al. 2001; Mina and Sledage 2006).

An Important effector mechanism of mAbs appears to be perturbation of signaling events that promote proliferation and survival of target cells. Some mAbs work by physically blocking the interaction between growth factor and its receptor, others by sterically hindering the receptor from assuming a conformation necessary for signaling (Sunada et al. 1986; Li et al. 2005). Virtually every clinically effective, unconjugated mAb perturbs signaling that promotes the proliferation and survival of the targeted cell population (Adams and Weiner 2005).

To compensate for the lack of potency of mAbs, countless methods have been devised to use monoclonals as targeting molecules that carry toxic payloads such as conjugated radioisotopes, toxins, and prodrug-converting enzymes (Wu and Senter 2005). While these approaches marginally increase the potency of monoclonals, they add significant manufacturing and quality-control costs and increase the regulatory hurdle by adding serious nonspecific toxicity. More recently, manipulations of Fc-domain structure have been described that customize antibody clearance and interaction with cellular Fc-receptors (Shields et al. 2001; Ghetie and Ward 2000; Umana et al. 1999). These modifications appear to increase the potency of monoclonals in in vitro assays, but so far there is no evidence that such modifications will increase clinical efficacy.

Currently, most polyclonal antibody (pAb) preparations for human use are derived from human plasma (Casadevall et al. 2004). Such polyclonals (intravenous immunoglobulin, IVIg) are used to prevent and treat many virus infections including rabies, cytomegalovirus, measles, rubella, hepatitis A and B, and varicella; IVIg therapy is indicated for post-exposure prophylaxis, and treatment of acute infections in immunosuppressed patients and newborns. However, despite its clinical success, the supply of IVIg is limited and large quantities must be administered because of the product's low specific activity (in general, neutralizing titers are 1:4 to 1:8). In contrast, polyclonal antisera taken from hyperimmunized animals have high specific activity but upon repeated usage in humans inflict significant side effects. Despite these limitations pAbs from hyperimmunized sheep, horses, and rabbits are the treatment of choice for venoms, bacterial toxins, and organ rejection (Casadevall et al. 2004; Casadevall 2002; Burton et al. 2006; Okum et al. 2006; Knight et al. 2006; Webster et al. 2006; Rainey and Young 2004). Spider or snake venoms contain a large number of diverse poisonous compounds that cannot be neutralized by a single mAb. Similarly, a number of bacteria produce several virulence factors that cannot be neutralized with a single antibody. In addition, it has been demonstrated that complexation of low molecular weight compounds, like botulinum neurotoxin or interleukins, with one or two mAbs actually prevents clearance and prolongs the half-life of the low molecular weight compound (Lu et al. 1995; Tomlinson and Zitener 1993; Finkelman et al. 1993; Sato et al. 1993; Debets and Savelkoul 1994; Mihara et al. 1991; Klein and Brailly 1995; Montero-Julian et al. 1994; Heremans et al. 1992; May et al. 1993). The minimum number of antibodies in an antigen–antibody complex that triggers rapid clearance of an antigen appears to be three. Therefore, effective elimination of venoms and toxins requires oligoclonal or polyclonal antibody preparations.

Another frequently used animal-derived pAb preparation comprises anti-T cell globulins (ATG) prepared in horses and rabbits (Burton et al. 2006; Okum et al. 2006; Knight et al. 2006; Webster et al. 2006). For the last 40 years rabbit ATG has been used for immunosuppression in organ graft recipients, and over 200,000 patients have been treated worldwide. The excellent safety profile of Thymoglobulin (Genzyme, Cambridge, MA) and Fresenius ATG (Fresenius Biotech, Graefelfing, Germany) demonstrates that rabbit IgG can be used safely in immunocompromised individuals.

Polyclonal antibodies from animals are also considered safe drugs if used nonchronically in healthy persons. Recently, the FDA approved Thymoglobulin and DigiFab (Protherics, Nashville, TN), polyclonal antibody preparations from rabbits and sheep, respectively. In addition, ten polyclonal antibody preparations from human plasma were approved in the last 5 years.

3 Overcoming Limitations of mAb Therapy

Devastating diseases such as cancer and infections with virulent pathogens are difficult to treat due to their complexity, multi-factorial etiology, and adaptivity. Therapies such as monoclonals directed against singularly defined targets fail when those targets change, evolve, and mutate. Such adaptive evolution is the bane of mono-specific drugs, which are quickly circumvented by resistant strains.

A well known example is Staphylococcus, which causes an ever increasing number of infections resistant to currently available antibiotics. Staphylococci elaborate a broad range of virulence factors that enable the organism to colonize, infect, and eventually cause disease in a variety of host tissues. Among these virulence factors are several adhesion molecules (MSCRAMMs) (Foster and Hook 1998; Simpson et al. 2003; Wann et al. 2000), capsular polysaccharides (O'Riordan and Lee 2004), extracellular toxins, hemolysins, superantigens (Ladhani 2003; Novick 2003; Schafer and Sheil 1995), protein A (Gomez et al. 2004), mediators of antibiotic resistance (Hiramatsu 2001; Srinivasan et al. 2002), proteases (Dubin 2002), lipases (Gotz et al. 1998), and formation of biofilm (Fowler et al. 2001; Rhode et al. 2001). While interference with any single one of these virulence factors results in some protection in animal models, effective therapy of infected humans most likely requires interference on several levels.

In cancer, development of multi-drug resistance is a common phenomenon (Vincent 2006; Fojo and Menefee 2005; Tulpule 2005; Vasir and Labhasetwar 2005; Vidal et al. 2004). With regards to the expression of particular cancer associated cell surface antigens there is a wide variation in expression levels between cancer cells of different patients (Golay et al. 2001). Cells expressing low levels of target antigen frequently escape mAb therapy and eventually rebound. For example, rituximab treatment has shown impressive remission rates in low-grade B cell lymphoma, but all patients develop resistance. For this reason, combination therapies of CD20 with chemotherapy are in use to prolong response rates (Hillmen 2004; Chow et al. 2002; Czuczman et al. 1999; Czuczman 1999; Vose et al. 2001).

One possible solution to address these issues is antibody therapy with a mixture of a limited number of mAbs (an oligoclonal antibody preparation, oAb) or with a polyclonal antibody preparation from serum (mixture of many antibodies, pAb). Such antibody preparations will be specific for several epitopes of one or several target molecules. Binding of antibodies to several epitopes of one or several antigens will increase the concentration of surface bound antibody and trigger antibody-dependent effector functions more effectively than a single monoclonal. As a consequence, cells with low expression levels of target antigens may be eliminated effectively. In addition, oAbs or pAbs may allow elimination of heterogeneous cell populations and reduce selection of escape mutations.

The synergistic effect of mixtures of mAbs has been demonstrated in clinical trials, where rituximab (anti-CD20) therapy was combined with anti-CD19 or anti-CD22 therapy (Sapra and Allen 2004; Herrera et al. 2003; Stein et al. 2004; Leonard et al. 2005). Similarly, the potency of pAbs is well documented. Currently, polyclonal antibodies for human therapy are produced in horses (botulinum, snake venom), rabbits (anti-thymocyte), and humans (CMV, vaccinia, botulinum, HepA, and HepB). Recently a number of in vivo and in vitro studies elucidating the mechanism of action of ATG (anti-thymocyte rabbit globulin: Thymoglobulin) have been performed (Michallet et al. 2003; Preville et al. 2001; Bonnefoy-Berard and Revillard 1996; Bonnefoy-Berard et al. 1994; Beiras-Fernandez et al. 2006). The results demonstrated that ATG eliminated not only T cells but also B cells and macrophages through complement fixation, ADCC, and induction of apoptosis. In addition, it stimulated proliferation of regulatory T cells. A clinical trial comparing Thymoglobulin with basiliximab (a monoclonal anti-CD25 antibody) for induction immunosuppression in cadaveric renal transplant recipients demonstrated 2.8 times lower acute rejection frequency in the ATG arm at a mean follow up of 9.8+/-3.9 months, while adverse events were similar in both groups (Brennan et al. 2006).

4   Limitations of Oligoclonal Antibody Therapy

Even though oAb (mixture of a few mAbs) therapy appears to be an attractive strategy to overcome some of the limitations of mAb therapy, there are several stumbling blocks in the realization of this approach. In particular, these impediments are the cost of development of several mAbs for the same indication, increased immunogenicity, lower safety, and difficult repeat dosing due to different pharmacokinetics and pharmacodynamics of mAbs.

The manufacturing of oAbs requires production of several mAbs contained in the mixture. The development and manufacturing of mAbs is labor intensive and, therefore, costly. In order to minimize production cost it has been proposed to combine cell lines expressing different mAbs in a single fermentor. A recent publication described the production of such an oligoclonal antibody preparation by co-cultivation of transfected CHO cell lines expressing various mAbs against Rhesus factor (Wiberg et al. 2006). Comparison of several independent production runs demonstrated consistent levels of individual mAbs in the culture broth. However, even though recombinant DNA encoding the various mAbs was integrated into the genome of CHO cells site-specifically using the FRT/Flp-In recombinase system, expression of individual mAbs differed substantially, with an up to 30-fold difference between lowest and highest producers. Currently, it is unclear if the observed differences in mAb expression are due to variation in transcription or in protein translation. These results suggest that production of oligoclonal antibody preparations will require fermentation of individual mAb-producing cell lines and subsequent mixing.

Due to the limited number of mAbs in oligoclonal antibody preparations, each individual antibody in the mixture should be efficacious and safe. Therefore, efficacy and safety has to be demonstrated for each individual antibody as well as for the oAb mixture. As a consequence, the cost of preclinical development of oAbs will be substantially higher and longer than the development of a single mAb.

Safety of mAb therapy is dependent on mechanism-dependent and mechanism-independent toxicities. Mechanism-independent toxicities relate to the occasional hypersensitivity reactions caused by a protein containing xenogeneic sequences and contaminants. Humanization of animal-derived mAbs allowed the generation of chimeric and humanized antibodies which cause sensitization of a low number of treated patients. Nevertheless, the immunogenicity problem is not eliminated with removal of all xenogeneic sequences (Pendley et al. 2003; Hwang and Foote 2005). The idiotype of a mAb, even a so-called fully human antibody, may be recognized as foreign by the immune system of certain patients. Currently available data indicate that even therapy with fully human mAb results in immune responses in up to 15% of treated patients. Sensitization of patients results in the formation of human anti-mAb antibodies that neutralize and/or eliminate circulating mAb, making it difficult or impossible to achieve therapeutic levels. In the worst case, hypersensitivity is sufficiently severe to require aggressive treatment of symptoms and discontinuation of therapy. Based on the observation that idiotypes of mAbs cause sensitization in certain patients it appears likely that oAbs containing several mAbs will cause sensitization of a higher number of patients than single mAb therapy.

Mechanism-dependent toxicities result from binding of the antibody to its target. Examples include cardiac toxicity occurring during trastuzumab antibody therapy of breast cancer, because heart tissue expresses low levels of anti-Her2/neu (Slamon et al. 2001). Treatment with rituximab can cause a profound first-dose toxicity related to the rapid lysis of normal and malignant B cells expressing CD20 (Byrd et al. 1999). Cetuximab therapy causes significant skin eruptions that are based on epidermal growth factor receptor (EGFR) expression in the skin (Robert et al. 2001; Herbst and Langer 2002). Bevacizumab, targeting vascular endothelial growth factor (VEGF) can induce hypertension, bleeding, thrombosis, or proteinuria (Hurwitz et al. 2004). Anti-CD3 antibodies or agonistic anti-CD28 antibodies can cause a severe cytokine release of activated cells. Based on these observations, it appears likely that mechanism-dependent toxicity of oAbs will be more frequent than such toxicities of single mAbs.

Besides differences in immunogenicity, mAbs display substantially different pharmacokinetics and pharmacodynamics (Lobo et al. 2004). The half-life of currently approved mAbs differs between 0.3 and 27 days. To complicate things further the pharmacokinetics of a particular mAb can vary substantially between patients. For example, the half-life of trastuzumab has been shown to vary between 2.7 and 10 days. These differences are influenced by a number of factors including the target antigen, binding-affinity, Fc-receptor binding, and immunogenicity. Therefore, mAbs in an oAb preparation are expected to display different pharmacokinetics and pharmacodynamics, and repeat dosing of oAbs to maintain a consistent effective antibody concentration of each individual antibody in a patient will be difficult.

The clinical development of antibody therapies requires a demonstration of safety and efficacy in human patients. Due to differences in toxicity and pharmacokinetics, it is expected that the safety of each individual mAb needs to be demonstrated in humans. The medical need of oAb therapy implies that mAb therapy in a particular patient population is rather ineffective. Therefore, a demonstration of efficacy of each individual mAb in the oAb mixture will be difficult and require large clinical studies.

Taken together, oAb therapy is expected to be more effective than mAb therapies, but in all likelihood also more expensive, more immunogenic, and less safe.

5   The Future of Antibody Therapy: Polyclonal Antibodies

Like oAbs, pAbs from human or animal serum have been shown to be effective because they can address multiple targets over heterogeneous cell populations and therefore have expanded utility in treating diseases not effectively treated today with mAbs. Currently, polyclonal antibodies for human therapy are produced in horses (botulinum, snake venom), rabbits (anti-thymocyte), and humans (i.e., CMV, vaccinia, botulinum, HepA, and HepB). Polyclonals purified from human plasma have low potency, and large amounts of pAb are required to treat and/or prevent human diseases effectively. On the other hand, pAb produced from animals have high titers (100- to 1,000-fold higher than human plasma-derived specialty IVIg preparations) and manufacturing costs are similar to mAbs. Due to high antigen-specific antibody titers, dosing of animal-derived IgG in hyperimmunized animals is similar to mAb dosing requirement (0.1–3 mg/kg). A significant advantage of pAbs is their lack of immunogenicity. Repeated administration of polyclonal antibody preparations derived from human plasma (IVIg) did not result in detectable anti-idiotypic antibody responses or other anti-human responses (Andresen et al. 2000). Similarly, anti-idiotypic antibodies could not be detected in patients treated with a rabbit-derived pAb (Thymoglobulin) (Regan et al. 1997). This is probably due to the low concentration of each individual antibody expressing one idiotype in the pAb.

To produce large quantities of safe, nonimmunogenic polyclonal antibodies of high avidity, it is necessary to move from human production to genetically engineered animals. The development of transgenic mice that produce human antibodies was a breakthrough and permitted the production of human antibodies of a desired specificity (Lonberg 2005). However, to produce commercial levels of human polyclonal antisera from transgenic animals, it is necessary to use a larger species such as cows, pigs, chickens, or rabbits.

The selected animal must produce sufficient volumes of antiserum to meet supply requirements. In addition, the animals must have a short breeding cycle to enable rapid scale-up and to allow the use of a large number of animals for antibody production. To obtain high batch-to-batch consistency of antibody specificities and titers, it is necessary to harvest sera for a limited period of time after immunization (a few weeks) and to pool sera from a large number of animals (>100). Rabbits have a gestation period of 28 days, conceive with every mating, have an average litter size of eight, and reach sexual maturity at the age of 5 months. As a consequence, a pair of sexually mature rabbits can be expanded to more than 500 animals within 1 year, corresponding to a biomass of 2,500 kg (approximately the mass of three mature cows). These characteristics allow the production of polyclonal antibodies by using a large number of rabbits per batch. In contrast, the long generation times of large farm animals (e.g., 2.5 year for cows), and the small number of offspring per conception, necessitate the extended use of a limited number of these larger animals for antibody production. The use of an extended bleeding schedule, coupled with the necessity of booster injections to maintain sufficient levels of specific antibodies, will result in variation of antibody specificities over time and in a tendency to oligoclonality.

The animal should be of a size and temperament to allow for ease of handling and maintenance of proper sanitation. Optimally, the animal should be an accepted source of GMP-produced therapeutics by the FDA. Currently, rabbits are the only species that meet these criteria. Several contractors in the United States and Europe currently produce GMP polyclonal antibodies from rabbits. The products include, for example, Thymoglobulin and Fresenius ATG, which are sold in the United States and Europe and consist of clinical-grade rabbit polyclonal preparations produced under GMP conditions. The use of these products in over 200,000 patients worldwide has demonstrated the excellent safety profile of therapeutic rabbit IgG in humans.

Based in part on the perceived notion that the cost of therapeutic polyclonals will be lower with the large blood volumes of cows and pigs, these animals are being used for genetic engineering. However, it is important to understand that the costs of the downstream manufacturing activities for therapeutic antibodies (purification, sterility, quality control, and final fill) are very similar regardless of the antibody source, and these constitute more than 90% of the final manufacturing cost.

For the effective expression of a human antibody repertoire in a farm animal it is important to consider species-specific aspects of B cell development and antibody diversification. Generally, all vertebrates start the creation of the primary antibody repertoire by recombining V, D, and J gene segments. In mice and humans this step results in considerable diversity as hundreds of VDJ genes are randomly recombined and genes are imprecisely joined together. In most other vertebrates, including rabbits, chickens, and cows, this first step of VDJ recombination does not lead to significant diversity because only a limited number of V genes are employed. To enhance diversity of the primary repertoire, these animals use a second step to modify antigen-binding regions through templated and/or nontemplated (hypermutation) mutational processes. The process of gene conversion transfers sequence information encoded (i.e., templated nucleotide substitutions) in upstream V genes to the rearranged exons (Fig. 1). A rearranged V gene undergoes several gene-conversion events during B cell development, resulting in changes to each of the antigen-binding sites or CDRs. Even though these processes are different between rabbits and humans, both mechanisms create a similar magnitude of antibody diversity (Knight and Crane 1994; Lanning et al. 2000; Weill and Reynaud 1996).

It is notable that gene conversion of endogenous antibody genes is not used for the generation of the antibody repertoire in humans and rodents. Based on these differences, one may speculate that the placement of an entire human immunoglobulin locus into a gene-converting animal may not result in sufficient antibody diversification for the production of high-titer, high-affinity antibodies, since neither gene conversion nor recombination/hypermutation will occur in an efficient manner.

Another important difference to consider is in immunophysiology. In mice and humans the fetal liver, omentum, and bone marrow serve as primary sites for B cell development, and the process of immunoglob-

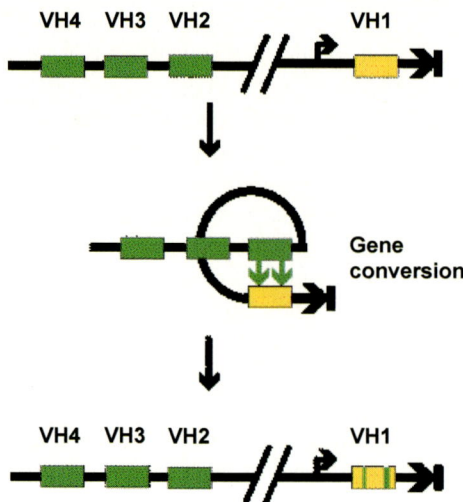

Fig. 1. Schematic representation of gene conversion. In gene conversion, DNA sequences from upstream V gene segments are introduced into the rearranged V gene. Homology between V genes is required for gene conversion to occur. Due to conserved framework regions, most changes are in the CDR regions of the rearranged V gene. Therefore gene conversion mimics "CDR grafting"

ulin gene rearrangement appears to occur throughout life. In rabbits diversification by gene conversion occurs in the appendix and other gut-associated lymphoid tissue, in chickens it occurs in the bursa of Fabricius, and in cows in spleen. Rearrangement of Ig genes stops in the chicken at hatching and diminishes after birth in rabbits, cows, and sheep.

Several companies are currently working on the generation of genetically engineered large animals for the production of human polyclonal antibodies: Hematech on cows, Revivicor on pigs, Origen on chicken, and Therapeutic Human Polyclonals (THP) on rabbits.

Fig. 2. Schematic representation of THP's approach to express human antibodies in animals. Only coding regions in the rabbit immunoglobulin gene were replaced with the corresponding human gene elements

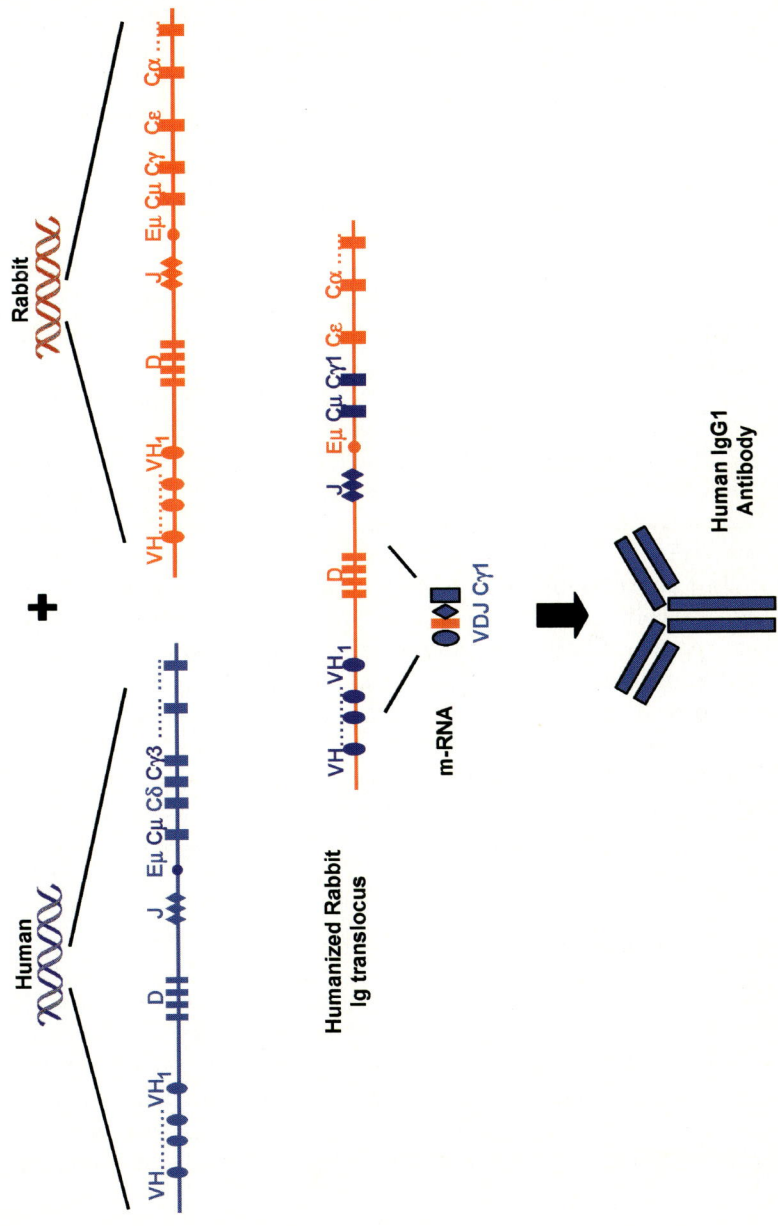

Hematech (a wholly owned subsidiary of Kirin Brewery Co.) generated transgenic cows by nuclear transfer cloning of bovine primary fetal fibroblast transfected with a human artificial chromosome. Similar to observations in mice, the expression of human immunoglobulin in wild-type cows was low (<1 μg/ml) (Kuroiwa et al. 2002). This may be because the human immunoglobulin locus cannot compete effectively with the cow's endogenous loci. One may speculate that this is due to the fact that cows generate a diverse antibody repertoire by gene conversion. In the meantime cows with inactivated immunoglobulin heavy chain loci have been generated (Kuroiwa et al. 2004), but, as of today, expression levels of human antibodies in knockout cows have not been reported.

A different approach has been developed by THP for the genetic engineering of rabbits. This novel approach is based on the humanization of rabbit immunoglobulin loci through replacement of protein coding rabbit DNA sequences with corresponding human counterparts while leaving the endogenous regulatory and antibody-production machinery intact (Fig. 2).

This human–animal translocus is expected to be a substrate for enzymes involved in DNA repair by gene conversion to support production and diversification of high-titer, high-affinity antibodies in gene-converting animals. The rabbit is particularly well suited for this approach because B cell immunology and antibody production in rabbits have been extensively characterized.

THP has validated this approach by successfully creating transgenic rabbits that produce humanized light chains and heavy chains. In these animals IgG levels of up to 2 mg/ml have been observed.

6   Conclusion

Antibodies have been used successfully as therapeutics for over 100 years. The successful development of therapeutic human(ized) mAbs in the last 20 years has demonstrated the potency of mAbs but also revealed some of their limitations. Studies in animals and humans demonstrated that it is possible to overcome some of these limitations using mixtures of antibodies. Combination therapy with several mAbs appears to be limited by the high cost of development of several mAbs for the same indication. In addition, such mixtures are expected to be more immunogenic and less safe than mAbs. Differences in pharmacokinetics and pharmacodynamics of individual mAbs make repeat dosing of such mixtures difficult. Such limitations can be overcome using pAbs.

Novel technologies are being developed for the production of human pAbs in genetically engineered animals. Immunization of such animals should allow the production of effective and safe high-titer antibody preparations for the treatment of infectious diseases, cancer, and autoimmunity.

References

Adams GP, Weiner LM (2005) Monoclonal antibody therapy of cancer. Nat Biotechnol 23:1147–1157

Andresen I, Kovarik JM, Spycher M, Bolli R (2000) Product equivalence study comparing the tolerance, pharmacokinetics and pharmacodynamics of various human immunoglobulin-G formulations. J Clin Pharmacol 40:722–730

Badger C, Anasetti C, Davis J, Bernstein I (1987) Treatment of malignancy with unmodified antibody. Pathol Immunopathol Res 6:419–434

Beiras-Fernandez A, Chappell D, Hammer C, Thein E (2006) Influence of polyclonal anti-thymocyte globulins upon ischemia-reperfusion injury in a nonhuman primate model. Transpl Immunol 15:273–279

Bonnefoy-Berard N, Revillard JP (1996) Mechanisms of immunosuppression induced by antithymocyte globulins and OKT3. J Heart Lung Transplant 15:435–442

Bonnefoy-Berard N, Genestier L, Flacher M, Rouault JP, Lizard G, Mutin M, Revillard JP (1994) Apoptosis induced by polyclonal antilymphocyte globulins in human B-cell lines. Blood 83:1051–1059

Brennan DC, Daller JA, Lake KD, Cibrik D, Del Castillo D, et al (2006) Rabbit anti-thymocyte globulin compared to basiliximab for induction in renal transplantation. New England J Med 355:1967–1977

Buchwald UK, Pirofski L (2003) Immune therapy for infectious diseases at the dawn of the 21st century: the past, present and future role of antibody therapy, therapeutic vaccination and biological response modifiers. Curr Pharm Des 9:945–968

Burton CM, Andersen CB, Jensen AS, Iversen M, Milman N, Boesgaard S, Arendrup H, Eliasen K, Carlsen J (2006) The incidence of acute cellular rejection after lung transplantation: a comparative study of anti-thymocyte globulin and daclizumab. J Heart Lung Transplant 25:638–647

Byrd JC, Waselenko JK, Maneatis TJ, Murphy T, Ward FT, Monahan BP, Sipe
    MA, Donegan S, White CA (1999) Rituximab therapy in hematologic ma-
    lignancy patients with circulating blood tumor cells: association with in-
    creased infusion-related side effects and rapid blood tumor clearance. J Clin
    Oncol 17:791–795
Cartron G, Dacheux L, Salles G, Solal-Celigny P, Bardos P, Colombat P, Watier
    H (2002) Therapeutic activity of humanized anti-CD20 monoclonal anti-
    body and polymorphism in IgG Fc receptor FcgammaRIIIa gene. Blood
    99:754–758
Casadevall A (2002) Passive antibody administration (immediate immunity) as
    a specific defense against biological weapons. Emerg Infect Dis 8:833–841
Casadevall A, Scharff MD (1994) Serum therapy revisited: animal models of
    infection and development of passive antibody therapy. Antimicrob Agents
    Chemother 38:1695–1702
Casadevall A, Scharff MD (1995) Return to the past: the case for antibody-
    based therapies in infectious diseases. Clin Infect Dis 21:150–161
Casadevall A, Dadachova E, Pirofski LA (2004) Passive antibody therapy for
    infectious diseases. Nat Rev Microbiol 2:695–703
Chow KU, Sommerlad WD, Boehrer S, Schneider B, Seipelt G, Rummel MG,
    Hoelzer D, Mitrou PS, Weidmann E (2002) Anti-CD20 antibody (IDEC-
    C2B8, rituximab) enhances efficacy of cytotoxic drugs on neoplastic lym-
    phocytes in vitro; the role of cytokines, complement and caspases. Haema-
    tologica 87:33–43
Church AC (2003) Clinical advances in therapies targeting the interleukin-2
    receptor. QJM 96:91–102
Czuczman MS (1999) CHOP plus rituximab chemoimmunotherapy of indolent
    B-cell lymphoma. Semin Oncol 26:88–96
Czuczman MS, Grillo-Lopez AJ, White CA, Saleh M, Gordon L, LoBuglio
    AF, Jonas C, Klippenstein D, Dallaire B, Varns C (1999) Treatment of pa-
    tients with low-grade B-cell lymphoma with the combination of chimeric
    anti-CD20 monoclonal antibody and CHOP chemotherapy. J Clin Oncol
    17:268–276
Debets R, Savelkoul HF (1994) Cytokine antagonists and their potential thera-
    peutic use. Immunol Today 15:455
Dubin G (2002) Extracellular proteases of Staphylococcus spp. Biol Chem
    383:1075–1086
Finckh A, Simard JF, Duryea J, Liang MH, Huang J, Daneel S, Forster A,
    Gabay C, Guerne PA (2006) The effectiveness of anti-tumor necrosis factor
    therapy in preventing progressive radiographic joint damage in rheumatoid
    arthritis: a population-based study. Arthritis Rheum 54:54–59

Finkelman FD, Madden KB, Morris SC, Holmes JM, Boiani N, Katona IM, Maliszewski CR (1993) Anti-cytokine antibodies as carrier proteins: prolongation of in vivo effects of exogenous cytokines by injection of cytokine-anti-cytokine antibody complexes. J Immunol 151:1235–1244

Fojo AT, Menefee M (2005) Microtubule targeting agents: basic mechanism of multidrug resistance (MDR). Semin Oncol 32:S3–8

Foster TJ, Hook M (1998) Surface protein adhesins of Staphylococcus aureus. Trends Microbiol 6:484–488

Fowler VG Jr, Fey PD, Reller LB, Chamis AL, Corey GR, Rupp ME (2001) The intercellular adhesin locus ica is present in clinical isolates of Staphylococcus aureus from bacteremic patients with infected and uninfected prosthetic joints. Med Microbiol Immunol (Berl) 189:127–131

Ghetie V, Ward ES (2000) Multiple roles for the major histocompatibility complex class I-related Fc receptor RcRn. Annu Rev Immunol 18:739–766

Golay J, Lazzari M, Facchinetti V, Bernasconi S, Borleri G, Barbui T, Rambaldi A, Introna M (2001) CD20 levels determine the in vitro susceptibility to rituximab and complement of B-cell chronic lymphocytic leukemia: further regulation by CD55 and CD59. Blood 98:3383–3389

Gomez MI, Lee A, Reddy B, Muir A, Soong G, Pitt A, Cheung A, Prince A (2004) Staphylococcus aureus protein A induces airway epithelial inflammatory responses by activating TNFR1. Nat Med 20:842–848

Gotz F, Verheij HM, Rosenstein R (1998) Staphylococcal lipases: molecular characterization, secretion, and processing. Chem Phys Lipids 93:15–25

Herbst R, Langer C (2002) Epidermal growth factor receptors as a target for cancer treatment: the emerging role of IMC-C225 in the treatment of lung and head and neck cancers. Semin Oncol 29:27–36

Heremans H, Dillen C, Put W, Damme JV, Billiau A (1992) Protective effect of anti-interleukin (IL)-6 antibody against endotoxin, associated with paradoxically increased IL-6 levels. Eur J Immunol 22:2395–2401

Herrera L, Yarbrough S, Ghetie V, Aquino DB, Vitetta ES (2003) Treatment of SCID/human B cell precursor ALL with anti-CD19 and anti-CD22 immunotoxins. Leukemia 17:334–338

Hillmen P (2004) Advancing therapy for chronic lymphocytic leukemia—the role of rituximab. Semin Oncol 31:22–26

Hiramatsu K (2001) Vancomycin-resistant Staphylococcus aureus: a new model of antibiotic resistance. Lancet Infect Dis 1:147–155

Holliger P, Hudson PJ (2005) Engineered antibody fragments and the rise of the single domains. Nat Biotechnol 23:1126–1136

Hoogenboom HR (2005) Selecting and screening recombinant antibody libraries. Nat Biotechnol 23:1105–1116

Hurwitz H, Fehrenbacher L, Novotny W, Cartwright T, Hainsworth J, Heim W, Berlin J, Baron A, Griffing S, Holmgren E, Ferrara N, Fyfe G, Rogers B, Ross R, Kabbinavar F (2004) Bevacizumab plus irinotecan, fluorouracil, and leucovorin for metastatic colorectal cancer. N Engl J Med 350:2335–2342

Hwang WY, Foote J (2005) Immunogenicity of engineered antibodies. Methods 36:3–10

Khazaeli MB, Conry RM, LoBuglio AF (1994) Human immune response to monoclonal antibodies. J Immunother 15:42–52

Klein B, Brailly H (1995) Cytokine-binding proteins: stimulating antagonists. Immunol Today 16:216

Knight KL, Crane MA (1994) Generating the antibody repertoire in rabbit. Adv Immunol 56:179–218

Knight RJ, Kerman RH, Zela S, Pdbielski J, Podder H, Van Buren CT, Katz S, Kahan BD (2006) Pancreas transplantation utilizing thymoglobulin, sirolimus and cyclosporine. Transplantation 81:1101–1105

Kohler G, Milstein C (1975) Continuous cultures of fused cells secreting antibody of predefined specificity. Nature 256:495–497

Kuroiwa Y, Kasinathan P, Choi YJ, Naeem R, Tomizuka K, Sullivan EJ, Knott JG, Duteau A, Goldsby RA, Osborne BA, Ishida I, Robl JM (2002) Cloned transchromosomic calves producing human immunoglobulin. Nat Biotechnol 20:889–894

Kuroiwa Y, Kasinathan P, Matsushita H, Sathiyaselan J, Sullivan EJ, Kakitani M, Tomizuka K, Ishida I, Robl JM (2004) Sequential targeting of the genes encoding immunoglobulin-mu and prion protein in cattle. Nat Genet 36:775–780

Ladhani S (2003) Understanding the mechanism of action of the exfoliative toxins of Staphylococcus aureus. FEMS Immunol Med Microbiol 39:181–189

Lanning D, Sethupathi P, Rhee KJ, Zhai SK, Knight KL (2000) Intestinal microflora and diversification of the rabbit antibody repertoire. J Immunol 165:2012–2019

Lee J, Fenton BM, Koch CJ, Frelinger JG, Lord EM (1998) Interleukin 2 expression by tumor cells alters both the immune response and the tumor microenvironment. Cancer Res 58:1478–1485

Leonard JP, Coleman M, Ketas J, Ashe M, Fiore JM, Furman RR, Niesvizky R, Shore T, Chadburn A, Horne H, Kovacs J, Ding CL, Wegener WA, Horak ID, Goldenberg DM (2005) Combination antibody therapy with epratuzumab and rituximab in relapsed or refractory non-Hodgkin's lymphoma. J Clin Oncol 23:5044–5051

Li S, Schmitz KR, Jeffrey PD, Wiltzius JJ, Kussie P, Ferguson KM (2005) Structural basis for inhibition of the epidermal growth factor receptor by cetuximab. Cancer Cell 7:301–311

Lobo ED, Hansen RJ, Balthasar JP (2004) Antibody pharmacokinetics and pharmacodynamics. J Pharm Sci 93:2645–2668

Lonberg N (2005) Human antibodies from transgenic animals. Nat Biotechnol 23:1117–1125

Lu ZY, Brailly H, Wijdenes J, Bataille R, Rossi JF, Klein B (1995) Measurement of whole body interleukin-6 (IL-6) production: prediction of the efficacy of anti-IL-6 treatments. Blood 86:3123–3131

May LT, Neta R, Moldawer LL, Kenney JS, Patel K, Sehgal PB (1993) Antibodies chaperone circulating IL-6. J Immunol 151:3225–3236

Michallet MC, Preville X, Flacher M, Fournel S, Genestier L, Revillard JP (2003) Functional antibodies to leukocyte adhesion molecules in antithymocyte globulins. Transplantation 75:657–662

Mihara M, Koishihara H, Fukui K, Ohsugi YY (1991) Murine anti-human IL-6 monoclonal antibody prolongs the half-life in circulating blood and thus prolongs the bioactivity of human IL-6 in mice. Immunology 74:55–59

Mina L, Sledage GW Jr (2006) Twenty years of systemic therapy of breast cancer. Oncology 20:25–32

Montero-Julian FA, Gautherot E, Wijdenes J, Klein B, Brailly H (1994) Pharmacokinetics of interleukin-6 during therapy with anti-interleukin-6 monoclonal antibodies: enhanced clearance of interleukin-6 by a combination of three anti-interleukin-6 antibodies. J Interferon Res 14:301–302

Novick RP (2003) Mobile genetic elements and bacterial toxinoses: the superantigen-encoding pathogenicity islands of Staphylococcus aureus. Plasmid 49:93–105

O'Riordan K, Lee JC (2004) Staphylococcus aureus capsular polysaccharides. Clin Microbiol Rev 17:218–234

Okum EJ, Perez-Tamayo RA, Higgins RS, Kasirajan V, Flattery M, Crowley S (2006) Administration of rabbit anti-thymocyte globulin during cardiopulmonary bypass: a novel approach to the highly sensitized cardiac transplant patient. J Heart Lung Transplant 25:608–610

Pendley C, Schantz A, Wagner C (2003) Immunogenicity of therapeutic antibodies. Curr Opin Mol Ther 5:172–179

Preville X, Flacher M, LeMauff B, Beauchard S, Davelu P, Tiollier J, Revillard JP (2001) Mechanisms involved in antithymocyte globulin immunosuppressive activity in a nonhuman primate model. Transplantation 71:460–468

Rainey GJ, Young JAT (2004) Antitoxins: novel strategies to target agents of bioterrorism. Nat Rev Microbiol 2:721–726

Regan J, Campbell K, van Smith L, Pouletty P, Schroeder TJ, Guttmann RD, Buelow R (1997) Characterization of anti-thymoglobulin, anti-ATGAM, and anti-OKT3 IgG antibodies in human serum with an 11-min ELISA. Transpl Immunol 5:49–56

Reichert JM, Dewitz MC (2006) Anti-infective monoclonal antibodies: perils and promise of development. Nat Rev Drug Discov 5:191–195

Reichert JM, Rosensweig CJ, Faden LB, Dewitz MC (2005) Monoclonal antibody successes in the clinic. Nat Biotechnol 23:1073–1078

Rhode H, Knobloch JK, Horstkotte MA, Mack D (2001) Correlation of Staphylococcus aureus icaADBC genotype and biofilm expression phenotype. J Clin Microbiol 39:4595–4596

Ringleb PA (2006) Thrombolytics, anticoagulants, and antiplatelet agents. Stroke 37:312–313

Robert F, Ezekiel MP, Spencer SA, Meredith RF, Bonner JA, Khazaeli MB, Saleh MN, Carey D, LoBuglio AF, Wheeler RH, Cooper MR, Waksal HW (2001) Phase I study of anti-epidermal growth factor receptor antibody cetuximab in combination with radiation therapy in patients with advanced head and neck cancer. J Clin Oncol 19:3234–3243

Sapra P, Allen TM (2004) Improved outcome when B-cell lymphoma is treated with combination of immunoliposomal anticancer drugs targeted to both the CD18 and CD20 epitopes. Clin Cancer Res 10:2530–2537

Sato TA, Widmer MB, Finkelman FD, Madani H, Jacobs CA, Grabstein KH, Maliszewski CR (1993) Recombinant soluble murine IL-4 receptor can inhibit or enhance IgE responses in vivo. J Immunol 150:2717

Schafer R, Sheil JM (1995) Superantigens and their role in infectious disease. Adv Pediatr Infect Dis 10:369–390

Shields RL, Namenuk AK, Hong K, Meng YG, Rae J, Briggs J, Xie D, Lai J, Stadlen A, Li B, Fox JA, Presta LG (2001) High resolution mapping of the binding site of human IgG1 for Fc gamma RI, Fc gamma RII, Fc gamma RIII and FcRn and designs of IgG1 variants with improved biding to the FC gamma R. J Biol Chem 276:6591–6604

Simpson KH, Bowden G, Hook M, Anvari B (2003) Measurement of adhesive forces between individual Staphylococcus aureus MSCRAMMs and protein-coated surfaces by use of optical tweezers. J Bacteriol 185:2031–2035

Slamon DJ, Leyland-Jones B, Shak S, Fuchs H, Paton V, Bajamonde A, Fleming T, Eiermann W, Wolter J, Pegram M, Baselga J, Norton L (2001) Use of chemotherapy plus a monoclonal antibody against HER2 for metastatic breast cancer that overexpresses HER2. N Engl J Med 344:783–792

Srinivasan A, Dick JD, Perl TM (2002) Vancomycin resistance in Staphylococci. Clin Microbiol Rev 15:430–438

Stein R, Zhengxing Q, Chen S, Rosario A, Shi V, Hayes M, Horak ID, Hansen HJ, Goldenberg DM (2004) Characterization of a new humanized anti-CD20 monoclonal antibody, IMMU-106, and its use in combination with the humanized anti-CD22 antibody, epratuzumab, for the therapy of non-Hodgkin's lymphoma. Clin Cancer Res 10:2868–2878

Sunada H, Magun BE, Mendelson J, MacLeod CL (1986) Monoclonal antibody against epidermal growth factor receptor is internalized without stimulating receptor phosphorylation. Proc Natl Acad Sci USA 83:3825–3829

Tomlinson A, Zitener HJ (1993) Enhancement of the biologic effects of interleukin-3 in vivo by anti-interleukin-3 antibodies. Blood 82:1133

Tulpule A (2005) Multidrug resistance in AIDS-related lymphoma. Curr Opin Oncol 17:466–468

Umana P, Jean-Maret J, Moudry R, Amstutz H, Bailey JE (1999) Engineered glycoforms of an antineuroblastoma IgG1 with optimized antibody-dependent cellular cytotoxic activity. Nat Biotechnol 17:176–180

Vasir JK, Labhasetwar V (2005) Targeted drug delivery in cancer therapy. Technol Cancer Res Treat 4:363–374

Vidal L, Attard G, Kaye S, De Bono J (2004) Reversing resistance to targeted therapy. J Chemother 26(4):7–12

Vincent M (2006) Tesmilifene may enhance breast cancer chemotherapy by killing a clone of aggressive, multi-drug resistant cells through its action on the p-glycoprotein pump. Med Hypotheses 66:715–7131

Vose JM, Link BK, Grossbard ML, Czuczman M, Grillo-Lopez A, Gilman P, Lowe A, Kunkel LA, Fisher RI (2001) Phase II study of rituximab in combination with CHOP chemotherapy in patients with previously untreated, aggressive non-Hodgkin's lymphoma. J Clin Oncol 19:389–397

Wann ER, Pohlmann-Dietze P, Steinhuber A, Chien YT, Manna A, van Wamel W, Cheung A (2000) Agr-independent regulation of fibronectin-binding protein(s) by the regulatory locus sar in Staphylococcus aureus. Mol Microbiol 36:230–243

Webster A, Pankhurst T, Rinaldi F, Chapman JR, Craig JC (2006) Polyclonal and monoclonal antibodies for treating acute rejection episodes in kidney transplant recipients. Cochrane Database Syst Rev 2:CD004756

Weill JC, Reynaud CA (1996) Rearrangement/hypermutation/gene conversion: when, where and why? Immunol Today 17:92–97

Weng WK, Levy R (2003) Two immunoglobulin G fragment C receptor polymorphisms independently predict response to rituximab in patients with follicular lymphoma. J Clin Oncol 21:3940–3947

Wiberg FC, Rasmussen SK, Frandsen TP, Rasmussen LK, Tengbjerg K, Coljee
    VW, Sharon J, Yang CY, Bregenholt S, Nielsen LS, Haurum JS, Tostrup
    AB (2006) Production of target-specific recombinant human polyclonal an-
    tibodies in mammalian cells. Biotechnol Bioeng 94:396–405
Wu AM, Senter PD (2005) Arming antibodies: prospects and challenges for
    immunoconjugates. Nat Biotechnol 23:1137–1146

Ernst Schering Foundation Symposium Proceedings

Editors: Günter Stock
Monika Lessl

Vol. 1 (2006/1): Tissue-Specific Estrogen Action
Editors: K.S. Korach, T. Wintermantel

Vol. 2 (2006/2): GPCRs: From Deorphanization
to Lead Structure Identification
Editors: H.R. Bourne, R. Horuk, J. Kuhnke, H. Michel

Vol. 3 (2007/3): New Avenues to Efficient Chemical Synthesis
Editors: P.H. Seeberger, T. Blume

Vol. 4 (2007/4): Immunotherapy in 2020
Editors: A. Radbruch, H.-D. Volk, K. Asadullah, W.-D. Doecke

Printing: Krips bv, Meppel
Binding: Stürtz, Würzburg